Pharmacy Management Software

for Pharmacy Technicians

| A WORKTEXT |

Pharmacy Management Software

for Pharmacy Technicians

| A WORKTEXT |

DAA Enterprises, Inc.
Brookline, Massachusetts

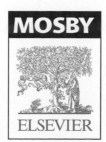

ELSEVIER

MOSBY
ELSEVIER

11830 Westline Industrial Drive
St. Louis, Missouri 63146

PHARMACY MANAGEMENT SOFTWARE   ISBN 13: 978-0-323-04958-0
FOR PHARMACY TECHNICIANS
Copyright © 2007 by Mosby, Inc., an affiliate of Elsevier Inc.

Notice

ISBN 13: 978-0-323-04958-0

Publishing Director: Andrew Allen
Executive Editor: Loren Wilson
Developmental Editor: Lynda Huenefeld
Publishing Services Manager: Julie Eddy
Project Manager: Andrea Campbell
Designer: Amy Buxton

Printed in the United States of America

Last digit is the print number: 9   8   7   6   5   4

Preface

Welcome to the exciting world of Pharmacy Technology! You have started on a journey into one of today's fastest-growing fields in health care. Whether you will end up working in a hospital pharmacy, a community pharmacy, one of the large pharmacy chain stores, or another location, the skills that you will gain from *Pharmacy Management Software for Pharmacy Technicians* will help prepare you well for your new career.

Pharmacy technicians are increasingly called upon to perform duties traditionally fulfilled by pharmacists. This is because of new federal regulations that now require pharmacists to spend more time with patients providing patient education. Because of the nature of the pharmacy technician's work, hands-on training is critically important in educational programs. This software package is designed to provide hands-on training and help you master the information and skills necessary to be a successful pharmacy technician. The various activities will challenge your knowledge, help further reinforce key concepts, and allow you to gauge your understanding of the subject matter studied in your pharmacy technician program.

Pharmacy Management Software for Pharmacy Technicians is a reliable and understandable resource written specifically for the pharmacy technician student. The worktext is divided into four sections—Retail Prescription Filling, Reports, Nursing Home, and Assessment. Each section guides you through the various tasks that pharmacy technicians are expected to be able to perform in a pharmacy setting.

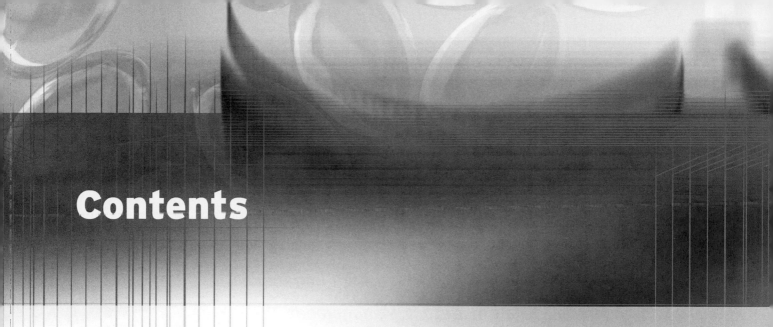

Contents

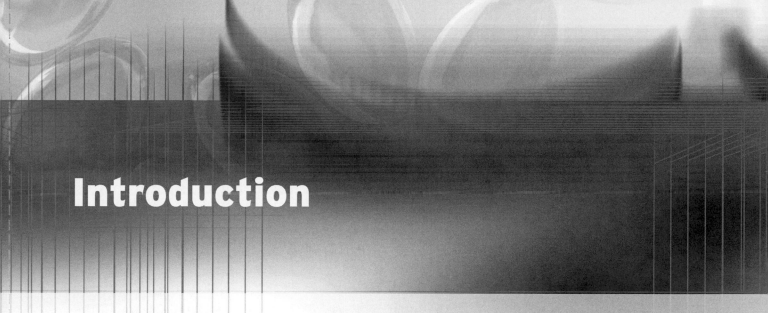

Introduction

Installation

Close all programs. Insert the CD labeled *Pharmacy Management Software for Pharmacy Technicians* into your CD-ROM drive. If Autorun is enabled on your system, this dialog box will be displayed. If Autorun is not enabled:

From the **Start** menu, select **Run.**

Type **D:\setup** (substitute the appropriate letter of your CD-ROM drive for D).

Press **Enter** or click on the 'Install' button to start installation.

The Installation Wizard will start to guide the rest of the setup. Click **Next** to view the End User License Agreement screen. Read the End User License Agreement carefully. Select **I accept** and click **Next.**

Select the destination folder. By default, the software is installed in C:\ Program Files\

Another dialog box prompts you for installation type. Select **Standalone or Server Installation.**

A final confirmation dialog box shows you all setup settings. Click **Next** to start copying the software from the CD to your computer. After all files have copied, click **Finish.** You may need to restart your computer to access the software after installation.

Please review the printed installation instructions provided with your CD-ROM.

Navigating Visual SuperScript

The Basics

Understanding the basics of software navigation is essential to your success in this course. If you are already familiar with Microsoft Windows applications, such as Word or Excel, you already have the basic navigation knowledge necessary. However, even if you are new to using a computer, you should be able to navigate the software after learning a few key concepts.

The first screen that you will see after installing the software is the main menu.

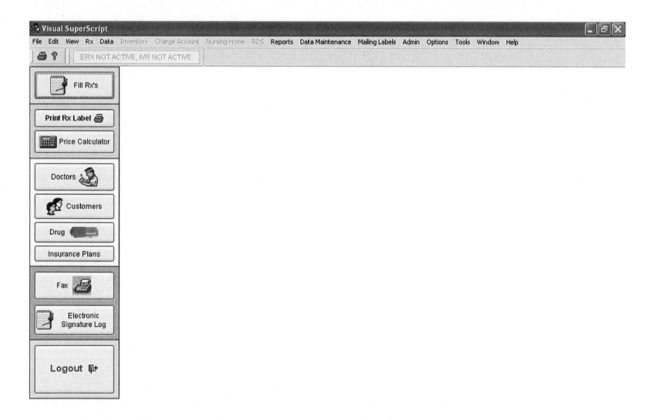

When you click on a menu choice that appears across the top of the main menu, you will see a drop-down list. Each menu choice on that drop-down list appears with one letter underlined. That letter represents a 'hot key' for that choice. Each item on the menu may be selected by pressing the Alt key and the corresponding hot key at the same time. For example, an Activity Summary may be selected from the **Reports** menu by pressing on **Alt** and the **A** key simultaneously.

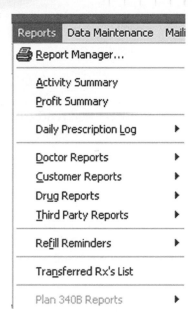

Of course, you may also select any menu option by moving the mouse pointer to it and clicking on it.

Note: Unless indicated otherwise, "Clicking the mouse" or "Clicking on it" means clicking the left mouse button once. On certain occasions you need to click the left button twice quickly. This is called "double clicking." Certain features of the program are accessed through menus that are displayed by clicking the right mouse button once. This is called "right clicking."

Objects, Icons, and Controls

You will interact with the software by using the various objects that appear on each form. Some objects appear as buttons with small pictures on them. These will be referred to as icons. Other objects appear as check-boxes, simple data entry areas referred to as text boxes or fields, and drop-down lists and combo boxes.

On most forms, there are multiple ways to enter data. There may be several text boxes and a few check boxes. The blinking cursor will provide you with a visual cue as to where you are in the form. To move from one space on a form to another, it is best to press the Tab key.

Text boxes

Text boxes are the most common objects that you will encounter. They are used to type in data or display numbers, such as names, DEA numbers, dates, etc. An example of text boxes are the Rx No., Disp Date, and the RPh Initials boxes on the Rx Processing form.

Rx No	
Dispense Date	/ /
RPh Initials	

Some text boxes may be 'read-only,' meaning they can only display information. Information cannot be added or changed in 'read-only' text boxes.

List boxes

List boxes are used when there are only certain responses you can use for a specific part of a form. Each list box has a downward small arrow next to it. You can see what choices you have for a text box by clicking on the downward arrow, and then clicking on the response of your choice. For example, when entering how a customer is going to pay for prescriptions, the user clicks on the arrow to the right of the pay type text box, and then selects either private or insurance from the dropdown list.

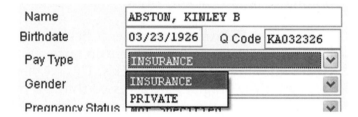

Combo boxes

Combo boxes are very similar to list boxes; however there are some differences. Visually, a combo box has a small icon next to it like a dropdown list, except the arrow has line below it. ⬓ The most important difference, however, is that the content in a combo box can be changed, unlike the content from a dropdown list. Combo boxes allow you to add, change, or remove information.

Icons

Icons, or buttons with pictures on them, appear throughout the software. However, you will mostly see icons on the File Navigation Toolbar that appears at the top of your screen.

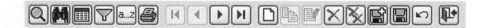

All of these buttons appear whenever a form designed for data entry is being used. These buttons are referred to as the navigation tools and the bar on which they appear is called the toolbar.

Each button has a picture that provides a clue about its function. A slightly more detailed explanation of the button's purpose may be obtained by moving the mouse pointer to a button and holding it there for several seconds. A small description of the button will appear.

The toolbar icons and corresponding purpose are as follows:

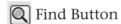 Find Button

This button is used to help find records.

![Locate icon] Locate Button

This button is used to locate records that meet certain criteria, such as families that live in a certain zip code.

![List icon] List Button

This button enables you to display the records in a file as a list.

![Filter icon] Filter Button

The filter button allows you to set filters so that only certain subsets of records are displayed. The filter function is similar to the locate function.

![Sort icon] Sort Button

The sort button allows you to select the order in which records are displayed.

![Print icon] Print Button

This button allowed you to print the record(s) that you are currently viewing.

![First icon] First Button

This button moves you back to the first record listed in a table.

![Prior icon] Prior Button

This button moves you to the prior record listed in a table.

▶ Next Button

This button moves you to the next record in a table.

▶| Last Button

This button moves you to the last record in a table.

□ New Button

Clicking this button displays a blank form to begin adding a new record.

▣ Copy Button

Clicking this button makes a copy of the current record and displays it for editing. This feature is handy when much of the information on a newly created record can be carried over from another record.

▣ Edit Button

Clicking this button allows you to make changes to a record.

✕ Delete Button

Clicking this button deletes the current record.

✕ Group Delete Button

This button allows a group of records that meet a certain criteria to be deleted.

▣ More Button

This button saves the current record and displays a blank form for adding a new record.

▣ Save Button

This button saves the current record.

↩ Cancel Button

This button cancels all changes made to the current record since the last time the record was saved.

▣ Close Button

This button closes the form.

RETAIL PRESCRIPTION FILLING

Adding a Physician or Prescriber to the Database

In this lab, you will:

- learn how to add a prescriber to the software database. Pharmacy software programs maintain a database of prescribers who have written the prescriptions that you fill in at the pharmacy.

Student Directions

Estimated completion time: 25 minutes

1. Read through the steps before performing the lab exercise on your computer.
2. After reading through the lab, perform the required steps using the sample prescription.
3. Complete the exercise at the end of the lab.

Dr. Robert P. Jones   office: 800/777-2211
109 10th Street   fax: 800/777-2212
Chicago, IL 60609

Patient Name:___Karen Anderson_____
Date:__3/7/06__
Address:_____

    Refill:____2 Times_____

    Rx: Adderal XR 10mg
        i q d
      #30

                                   Dr. Robert P. Jones
                                   AJ24681352

Product Selection Permitted   Dispense As Written

DEA NO.___AJ24681352_____
Address_____

HINT: Data entry fields are highlighted in blue when information is ready to be added.

Steps

Use the prescription above to complete the following steps.

1 Access the main screen of Visual SuperScript.

2 Click on the **Doctors** button located on the left side of the screen.

3 A dialog box entitled *Doctors* will pop up.

4 Click on the **New** icon located on the toolbar at the top of the dialog box.

5 The form is now ready for you to enter the prescriber information. Tab from one field to the next to enter information.

6 The **NAME** is a required field. It is 30 characters long, which should be adequate for most names. It is very important that names be entered consistently. Enter the prescriber name starting with the last name followed by a comma, one space, and then the first name. Middle initials or middle names may be appended to distinguish between two individuals having similar names.

> Enter *Jones, Robert*
> *Jones, Robert P.*

> **HINT:** Navigate through the form by using the **TAB** key.

7 The **CONTACT** field should contain the name of the person you usually talk to when you call the doctor's office for refill authorization. Being reminded of the person's name may help you add a personal touch to your phone calls.

> Enter *Nurse: Barb Little as contact.*

8 Enter the prescriber's **ADDRESS**.

> Enter *109 10th Street, Chicago, IL 60609.*

> **HINT:** After entering the street address, the software will take you to the **ZIP** field. Enter the zip and the city/state will fill in automatically.

9 Enter the prescriber's **PHONE** information. The fax number is particularly useful because Visual SuperScript can directly send faxes to the doctor's office when refill authorization is required.

Enter *800-777-2211.*

10 Tab to the **QUICK-CODE** field. Enter the prescriber's initials in the **QUICK-CODE** field. This field is designed to help retrieve data quickly when filling a prescription. For instance, in the future when filling a prescription written by Dr. Robert P. Jones, simply enter RJ in the **DOCTOR** field instead of typing out the entire physician name.

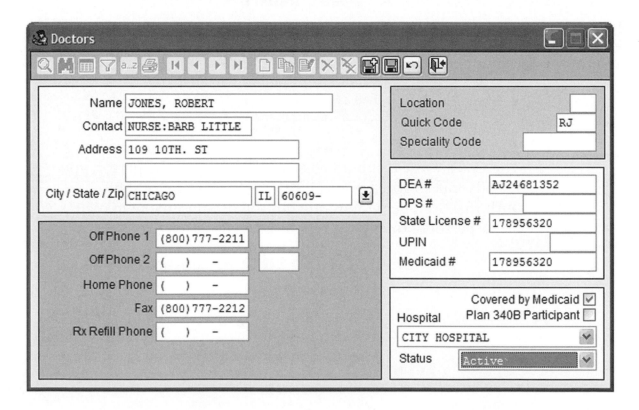

11 Enter the **LOCATION** and **SPECIALTY CODE** *only if required by your state*.

12 Enter the prescriber's **DEA** (Drug Enforcement Agency) number. The DEA number is necessary for any prescription that is written for a controlled substance. Additionally, many third-party payers require a DEA number as a means of identifying the prescriber. Note: A message box will appear indicating that the DEA number is invalid. Click "No" and continue to step 13. Valid DEA numbers will not be used in the exercises in this worktext.

Enter *AJ24681352*.

13 Enter the **DPS** (Department of Public Safety) number and the **UPIN** (Unique Physician Identification Number) number *only if required by your state.*

14 Enter the prescriber's **STATE LICENSE** number. Most states require the prescriber's **STATE LICENSE** number in order to process Medicaid claims. The prescriber's **STATE LICENSE** number may be found on the written prescription form. If the **STATE LICENSE** number is not provided, a phone call to the prescriber is necessary to find out this information.

Enter *178956320* as the STATE LICENSE number.

15 Enter the prescriber's **MEDICAID** number. In most cases, the **MEDICAID** number is the same as the **STATE LICENSE** number.

Enter *178956320* as the Medicaid number.

16 Keep the **COVERED BY MEDICAID** check box checked if the prescriber is authorized to write prescriptions for Medicaid-supported patients.

17 Click on the **ARROW** to the right of the **HOSPITAL** data entry field. This entry field designates the institutions that the prescriber has privileges at. Click on the correct hospital from the drop-down list.

Select *City Hospital*.

18   Click on the arrow to the right of the **Status** field. Click on **Active** from the drop-down list to indicate that the prescriber is in active practicing status.

19   Click on the **Save** icon [🖫] located at the top right of the toolbar.

20   Print the screen by using the **PrintScrn** option on your keyboard: Press the **PrintScrn** key, open a blank Word document, **Right Click** the blank Word document, and then select **Paste**.

21   Check with your instructor on the preferred method of submitting your work from step 19.

22   Return from the Word document to Visual SuperScript. Click the **Close** icon ✕ located at the top right of the toolbar.

Exercise

Scenario

Leslie Black presented the following prescription at your pharmacy. When inputting prescription data in the computer, you make note that Dr. Markus W. Paul is not in the pharmacy database.

Task

Following the steps from Lab 1: Adding a Physician or Prescriber to the Database, enter Dr. Markus W. Paul into the pharmacy database. Submit the added form for verification. Note: A message box will appear indicating that the DEA number is not valid. Click "No" and continue entering the prescriber's information.

Dr. Markus W. Paul
High Road South
Chicago, IL 60609

office: 800/669-9134
fax: 800/669-9130

Patient Name:___Leslie Black
Date:___1/7/2007
Address:_____

Refill:_____2 Times

Rx: Ativan 10mg
     prn
  #15

Dr. Markus W. Paul

AP24681352

Product Selection Permitted   Dispense As Written

DEA NO.___AP24681352
Address_____
State License # 37891

Advanced Exercise–Adding a Physician or Prescriber to the Database

LAB OBJECTIVES

In this lab, you will:

- apply skills learned in Lab 1: Adding a Physician or Prescriber to the Database. You will build on Lab 1 information and learn how to use the Find command, learn how to use the More command, and add new city and zip code information to the database.

Student Directions

Estimated completion time: 30 minutes

1. Read through the steps before performing the lab exercise on your computer.
2. After reading through the lab, perform the required steps to enter provider information.
3. Complete the exercise at the end of the lab.

Steps

1 Access the main screen of Visual SuperScript.

2 Click on the **Doctors** button located on the left side of the screen.

3 A dialog box entitled *Doctors* will pop up.

4 Click on the **Find** icon 🔍 located on the top left of the toolbar.

5 A dialog box entitled *Find* will pop up.

6 Enter the first three letters of the prescriber's last name in the **Name** field.

Enter *PET* for Dr. Larry Peterson.

7 Click on **OK** at the bottom of the dialog box.

8 If the prescriber is not in the database, a message will appear on the top right of the screen indicating *No Records Match Your Entry*.

9 Click on **Cancel** at the bottom of the *Find* dialog box. The dialog box will close out and the *Doctors* form will be active.

10 Click on the **New** icon located on the toolbar at the top of the dialog box.

11 The form is now ready for you to enter the prescriber information.

12 The **Name** is a required field. Enter the prescriber name starting with the last name followed by a comma, one space, and then the first name.

Enter *Peterson, Larry* for Dr. Larry Peterson.

13 The **Contact** field should contain the name of the person you usually talk to when you call the doctor's office for refill authorization.

Enter *Brandon* as the contact.

14 Enter the prescriber's **Address**.

Enter *11321 9th Street, Learning, IA 50115* as the address.

15 The city and zip code of the prescriber are not in the database. A pop-up table entitled *Zip* appears after entering the zip code.

16 Scroll through the *Zip* pop-up table to be certain that the desired zip code and city information is not in the database. Then click on **Cancel** at the bottom of the box. The *Zip* pop-up table will close out and the *Doctors* form will again be active.

> **HINT:** Use the vertical scroll bar located on the right side of the pop-up box to view zip code information.

17 To add the city and zip code to the database: right click the **ZIP CODE** data entry field.

    a. A pop-up menu will appear.

    b. Choose **ADD NEW** from the pop-up menu.

    c. A pop-up dialog box appears entitled *Zip Code*.

    d. Click **NEW.**

    e. Enter the prescriber zip code, city, and state abbreviation.

    f. Click on the **SAVE** icon located at the top right of the dialog box toolbar.

    g. Click on the **CLOSE** icon located at the top right of the toolbar.

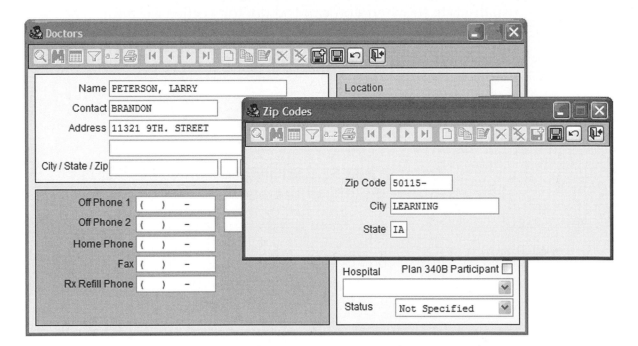

18 Press the **TAB** key to navigate through the address fields. The zip code information has now been added to the database. Verify that the correct zip code information has been added by clicking on the **COMBO-BOX ARROW** located to the right of the zip code data entry field. Note: If the zip code is in the database, the city/state fields will populate automatically.

19 A pop-up table appears entitled *Zip.*

20   Edit the zip code information if necessary by clicking on the **Edit** button located at the bottom of the pop-up box.

21   Click on the **OK** button when zip code information has been verified as correct.

22   Enter the prescriber's **Phone** information.

> **Enter *717/330-1990* extension *109* as the office phone.**
>
> **Enter *717/330-1991* as the fax number.**

23   Enter the prescriber's initials in the **Quick Code** field.

24   Enter the prescriber's **DEA** number. Enter the prescriber's **State License** number.

> **Enter the prescriber's Medicaid number.**
>
> **Enter *BP1234892* as the DEA number.**
>
> **Enter *11998822* as the State License number.**

25   Keep the **Covered by Medicaid** check box checked if the prescriber is authorized to write prescriptions for Medicaid-supported patients.

26   Click on the **Arrow** to the right of the Hospital field.

> **Select City Hospital.**

27 Click on the **Arrow** to the right of the **Status** field. Click on **Active** from the drop-down list to indicate that the prescriber is in active practicing status.

28 Click on the **Save** icon located at the top right of the dialog box toolbar.

29 Print the screen by using the **PrintScrn** option on your keyboard: Press the **PrintScrn** key, open a blank Word document, **Right Click** the blank Word document, and then select **Paste**.

30 Check with your instructor on the preferred method for submitting your work from step 28.

31 Click the **Close** icon located at the top right of the dialog box toolbar.

> **HINT:** When adding a group of prescribers at the same time, click on the **More** icon located on the top right of the dialog box toolbar. Use the **More** icon in place of the **Save** icon.

Exercise

Practice using the software data entry skills by entering the following prescriber information. Follow step 28 for each prescriber who is added to the database. Submit work when completed. Note: A message box will appear indicating that the DEA number is invalid. Click "No" and continue entering the prescriber's information.

Prescriber Information

1. Dr. Catelynn Judith
9608 Barroll Lane, Suite 333
Kensington, MD 20895
Phone: 301-962-3140
Fax: 301-962-3144
DEA: AJ1256948-012
State License/Medicaid: 77332
Contact: Jen

2. Dr. Emma Francis
2208 Colonial Acres Ct, Suite 444
Herndon, VA 20170
Phone: 703-430-3814
Fax: 703-430-3813
DEA: BF2368521
State License/Medicaid: 23569
Contact: Office Secretary

3. Dr. Markus Wayne
1812 Lincoln HWY, #52
Reston, VA 20190
Phone: 703-829-1100
Fax: 703-829-1111
DEA: AW7899562-134
State License/Medicaid: 96587
Contact: Judy

4. Dr. Jennifer Suz
1800 Lincoln HWY
Reston, VA 20194-1215
Phone: 703-829-1000
Fax: 703-829-1100
DEA: AS5478547
State License/Medicaid: 56921
Contact: Joe

5. Dr. Jacob Field
7500 Evans St.
Sterling, VA 20197
Phone: 703-571-2344

Fax: 703-571-2345
DEA: BF8527414
State License/Medicaid: 9863
Contact: Assistant—Ralph

6. Dr. Lucille Moore
7500 Evans St.
Pittsburgh, PA 15218
Phone: 412-571-2300
Fax: 412-571-2301
DEA: AM5698523
State License/Medicaid: 0023
Contact: none

7. Dr. Tom Pane
5121 Brightwood Rd., #110
Bethel Park, PA 15102
Phone: 412-835-4700
Fax: 412-835-4701
DEA: AP6985213
State License/Medicaid: 45698
Contact: Brenda

8. Dr. D. Kraft
11818 "F" Street
Omaha, NE 68137
Phone: 402-899-9911
Fax: 402-891-9912
DEA: AK2566326
State License/Medicaid: 23695
Contact: Brecken

9. Dr. I. Audubon
109 Eastside Dr.
Omaha, NE 68137
Phone: 402-891-5521
Fax: 402-891-5522
DEA: AA7856412
State License/Medicaid: 30256
Contact: Office Nurse

10. Prescriber Name:
Prescriber Address:
Phone:
Fax:
DEA:
State License/Medicaid:
Contact:

Adding a New Patient to the Database

In this lab, you will:

- learn how to add a new patient to the pharmacy software database

Student Directions

Estimated completion time: 45 minutes

1. Read through the steps before performing the lab exercise on your computer.

2. After reading through the lab, perform the required steps to enter patient information.

3. Complete the exercise at the end of the lab.

Steps

1 Access the main screen of Visual SuperScript.

2 Click on the **Customers** button located on the left side of the screen.

3 A dialog box entitled *Customers* will pop up.

4 Click on the **New** icon located on the dialog box toolbar.

5 The *Customers* dialog box contains four tabbed forms. Click on the tab entitled *Customer*.

6 The form is now ready to enter new patient information.

7 The **Name** is a required field and allows up to 30 characters. The recommended format is last name followed by a comma, a single space, first name, a single space, middle initial or name (if known). Example: Johnson, Linda P.

Enter *Mary E. Shedlock* as patient name.

HINT: To facilitate searching your database, it is very important that you follow the recommended format for entering names.

8 The format for entering the **Birthdate** is mm/dd/yyyy. Example: 03/03/1960 (do not enter as 3/3/1960).

9   **Q Codes** (Quick Codes) allow you to expedite the search for customers when filling prescriptions. Enter the patient's initials in this field. Enter *MS* for patient's initials.

10   **Pay type** is a very important field. It determines how prescriptions filled for this patient are priced and who is expected to pay for them. Two **Pay types** are permissible: Private and Insurance. Click on the **Arrow** located to the right of the **Pay type** data entry field. Select appropriate **Pay type**.

Select *Private*.

11   Click on the **Arrow** located to the right of the **Gender** data entry field. Select appropriate gender.

Select *Female*.

12   Click on the **Arrow** located to the right of the **Pregnancy Status** data entry field. Select appropriate status.

Select *Not pregnant*.

13   Click on the **Arrow** located to the right of the **Smoking** data entry field. Make appropriate selection.

Select *Not specified*.

14   The next data entry field is the **Patient Identification** field. The state government or the pharmacy may require additional patient identification information. Click on the **Arrow**. A drop-down list appears with patient ID choices. Click on the appropriate choice.

Select *Not specified* as the customer gave no other ID information.

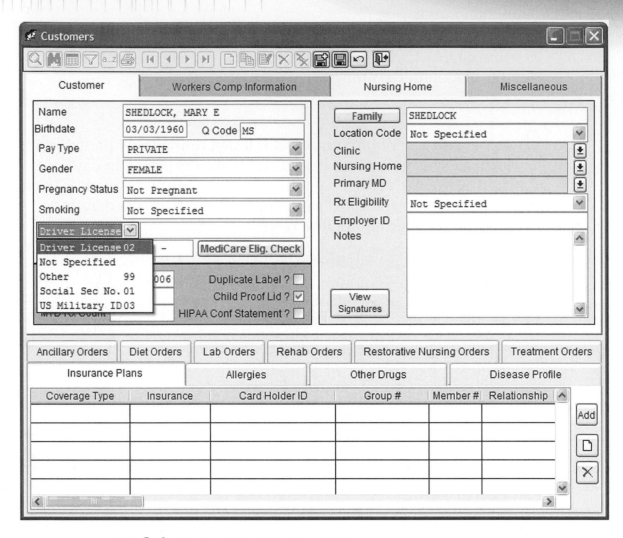

FIG **3-1**   Patient identification field.

15 The **First Visit Date** and **Last Visit Date** fields containing the date of the most recent prescription filled for the customer are automatically updated while filling prescriptions, so you do not have to enter any value in those fields.

16 The **MTD RX Count** field contains the month-to-date count of the number of prescriptions filled for this customer. This field is automatically updated while filling prescriptions. Therefore there is no need to manually enter a value in this field.

17 **Child-Proof Lid**: By default, this box will be checked for every customer that is added to the database because the law requires the use of such a lid unless specified otherwise. If a customer desires easy-open lids, make sure to uncheck this box. In that case, the words "EZ CAP" will appear on the hard-copy segment of the prescription label as a reminder.

18 **Duplicate Label**: Check this box if the customer requests two labels at the time the prescription for this patient is filled.

19 Tab to the **HIPAA Conf Statement** data entry field. Click in the check-off box to indicate that the patient has received HIPAA information.

20 Tab to the **Family** field. **Family** is a very important, required field. Customers are grouped into families, with each family having one individual designated as a **Family Head**. Each customer is linked to the family database by reference to the **Family Head**. Key in the name of the **Family Head** and press the **Tab** key. It may be necessary to first delete a **Family Head** name that the software automatically adds to this data entry field before adding the correct **Family Head** name.

Enter *Wright, Frank* as the **Family Head**.

21 A dialog box entitled *Family Head Lookup* appears on your screen. Click on the correct *Family Head Name* from the table. The name will now be highlighted in blue. Click on **OK** located at the bottom of the dialog box.

22 Click on the **Arrow** located to the right of the **Location Code** data entry field. Select **Home**.

23 Tab to the **Notes** field. In this field you can enter whatever information you want to store about the patient. The information will appear on the Prescription Processing Screen as a reminder when filling a prescription for this patient.

> **Enter for Notes: *Patient is hard of hearing in left ear.***

24 The bottom half of the *Customers* form contains various tabs. Click on the **Allergies** tab.

25 Click on the **Add a New Record** icon [D] located on the bottom right of the *Customers* form. An *Allergy Lookup* table pops up.

26 Key in the first two letters of the allergy in the **Allergy** data entry field. Use the scroll bar to select the appropriate allergy. Select the appropriate allergy by clicking on the allergy and then click on **OK**.

> **Key in *MO*. Select *morphine*. Click *OK*.**

27 Click on the **Other Drugs** tab. This grid contains information about other drugs that the patient is currently taking. These may be prescription drugs that were purchased from a different pharmacy, or they may be over-the-counter (OTC) drugs. For each such drug, a start date and estimated days of supply may also be entered. The purpose of recording this information is to check for possible drug interactions and duplicate ingredients and therapy.

28 Click on the **Add a New Record** icon located on the bottom right of the *Customers* form. Press the **Enter** key to access a list of drugs. A *Drug Name Lookup* table pops up.

29 Look up the drug by typing the name of the drug in the **Name** dialog box. Click on the desired drug to select. Click on **OK**.

Mary Shedlock began taking Lipitor
20 mg in 12/2006. She takes 1 tab q d.

30 Click on the **Disease Profile** tab. This grid contains a list of diseases the customer has been diagnosed for. The information contained in this grid is used to check for drug-disease contraindications each time a prescription is filled for the patient.

31 Click on the **Add a New Record** icon located on the bottom right of the *Customers* form. A red bar appears across the *Disease Profile* table.

32 Press the **F2** key. A *Disease Lookup* table pops up entitled *CFDBDX*.

33 Look up the disease by typing the first few letters of the name of the disease. Click on the desired disease to select. Click on **OK**.

Enter *hyperlipidemia* for the disease
high cholesterol.

34 Click on the **Save** icon located at the top right of the toolbar in the *Customers* dialog box.

35 Print the screen by using the **PrintScrn** option on your keyboard: Press the **PrintScrn** key, open a blank Word document, **Right Click** the blank Word document, and then select **Paste**.

36 Click the **Close** icon located at the top right of the toolbar.

> **HINT:** When adding a group of patients at the same time, click on the **More** icon located on the top right of the dialog box toolbar. Use the **More** icon in place of the **Save** icon.

Exercise

Practice using the software data entry skills by entering the following patient information. Submit work when completed.

Patient Information

Andrew J. Shedlock
DOB: 11/4/97
Allergies: penicillin
Private Pay
HOH: Frank Wright

Matthew Simon
DOB: 5/10/98
Allergies: sulfa (sulfa is listed in the allergy lookup with a group of meds)
Cash paying customer
HOH: Paul Simon

Colleen Duke
DOB: 8/10/50
Allergies: chocolate (chocolate will not be listed as a medication allergy under the **Allergy** tab; make a note of this food allergy in the notes field)
No insurance
HOH: Michael Duke
Wants easy-open lids
Takes Lipitor and HCTZ
Diagnosed with high cholesterol

Christina Rowen
DOB: 7/15/65
Allergies: tetracycline

Private pay
HOH: James Rowen
Takes OTC calcium with vit. D

Olivia Rose Rowen
DOB: 10/08/03
Allergies:
Private pay
HOH: James Rowen
Requests duplicate labels

David Henderson
DOB: 10/15/62
Allergies:
Cash paying customer
HOH: Gary Henderson
Takes metformin
Diagnosed with NIDDM

Charlie Henderson (male)
DOB: 6/12/01
Allergies:
No insurance
HOH: Gary Henderson

James White
DOB: 11/5/62
Allergies: penicillin, cephalosporins
Private pay
HOH: David R. White
Takes furosemide and baby ASA
Diagnosed with heart problems

Colleen Major
DOB: 3/10/60
Allergies: penicillin
Private pay
HOH: Samuel Malone
Requests no childproof caps
Takes Synthroid
Diagnosed with thyroid disease

Tom Roch
DOB: 9/4/50
Allergies: dairy products, codeine
No insurance
HOH: John Rogers
Takes Ativan, Wellbutrin, Bumex, and OTC daily vitamin
Diagnosed with depression

Tim Saba
DOB: 6/14/55
Allergies:
No insurance
HOH: Anne Saba

Dan Kaldor
DOB: 10/12/57
Allergies:
No insurance
HOH: James Kaldor

Joshua Graves
DOB: 4/15/57
Allergies: penicillin
Cash paying customer
HOH: Peter Graves

Ed Tedford
DOB: 12/2/56
Allergies:
Cash paying customer
HOH: Hazel Tedford
Takes diltiazem

Patient Name:
Address:
Phone:
DOB:
Allergies:
Other Medications:
Disease State:
HOH:

Advanced Exercise–Adding a New Patient to the Database

LAB OBJECTIVES

In this lab, you will:

- apply skills learned in Lab 3: Adding a New Patient to the Database
- build on Lab 3 information and learn how to use the ADD command, learn how to enter family head information, and learn how to enter insurance plan information for the patient
- learn what information is needed from the patient's insurance card when entering an insurance plan in the database
- review the procedure for adding zip codes, which was covered in Lab 2: Advanced Exercise–Adding a Physician or Prescriber to the Database

Student Directions

Estimated completion time: 1 hour

1. Read through the steps before performing the lab exercise on your computer.
2. After reading through the lab, perform the required steps to enter patient information.
3. Complete the exercise at the end of the lab.

Steps

1 Access the main screen of Visual SuperScript.

2 Click on the **Customers** button located on the left side of the screen.

3 A dialog box entitled *Customers* will pop up.

4 Click on the **Find** icon, which is located on the top left of the *Customers* dialog box toolbar.

5 A dialog box entitled *Customer Lookup* pops up. Enter the first letter of the customer's last name into the **Name** data entry field. Scroll through the *Customer Lookup* pop-up table to be certain that the customer is not in the database.

> **Enter S and scroll through table to see if Matthew Shultz is in the database.**

> **HINT:** Use the vertical scroll bar located on the right side of the pop-up box to view customer information.

6 The customer name is not located in the *Customer Lookup* table. Click on **Add** located at the bottom of the *Customer Lookup* dialog box.

7 The *Customers* dialog box appears. It contains four tabbed forms. Click on **Customer**.

8 The form is now ready to enter new patient information.

9 The **NAME** is a required field and allows up to 30 characters. The recommended format is last name followed by a comma, a single space, first name, a single space, and middle initial or name (if known). Example: Johnson, Linda P.

Enter *Matthew Shultz* as patient name.

> **HINT:** To facilitate searching your database, it is very important that you follow the recommended format for entering names.

10 The format for entering the **BIRTHDATE** is mm/dd/yyyy. Example: 05/10/1998 (do not enter as 5/10/1998).

Enter *05/10/1998* as the birthdate.

11 **Q CODES** (Quick Codes) allow you to expedite the search for customers when filling prescriptions. Enter the patient's initials in this field.

Enter *MS* for patient's initials.

12 **PAY TYPE** is a very important field. It determines how prescriptions filled for this patient are priced and who is expected to pay for them. Two **PAY TYPES** are permissible: Private and Insurance. Click on the **ARROW** located to the right of the **PAY TYPE** data entry field.

Select *Insurance*.

13 Click on the **ARROW** located to the right of the **GENDER** data entry field. Make appropriate selection. Select *Male*.

Select *Male.*

Note: The pregnancy status field locks automatically when "Male" is selected.

14 Click on the **ARROW** located to the right of the **SMOKING** data entry field. Make appropriate selection from the list.

Select *Not specified.*

15 The next data entry field is the **PATIENT IDENTIFICATION** field. The state government or the pharmacy may require additional patient identification information. Click on the **ARROW**. A drop-down list appears with patient ID choices. Click on the appropriate choice.

Select *Not specified.*

16 Tab to the blue section of the form. The **FIRST VISIT DATE** and the **LAST VISIT DATE** fields contain the date of the most recent prescription filled for the customer. It is automatically updated while filling prescriptions, so you do not have to enter any value in it manually.

17 The **MTD RX COUNT** field contains the month-to-date count of the number of prescriptions filled for this customer. It is automatically updated while filling prescriptions, so you do not have to enter any value in it manually.

18 **CHILD-PROOF LID:** By default, this box will be checked for every customer that is added to the database because the law requires the use of such a lid unless specified otherwise. If a customer desires easy-open lids, make sure to uncheck this box. In that case, the words "EZ CAP" will appear on the hard-copy segment of the prescription label as a reminder.

19 **DUPLICATE LABEL:** Check this box if the customer requests two labels at the time the prescription for this patient is filled.

20 Tab to the **HIPAA CONF STATEMENT** data entry field. Click in the check box ☑ to indicate that the patient has received HIPAA information.

21 Tab to the **FAMILY** data entry field. Press **ENTER**. A box entitled *Family Head Lookup* pops up. Click **ADD** to add the family head.

22 The *Families* dialog box appears on the screen. **FAMILY HEAD NAME** is a required field and allows up to 30 characters. The recommended format is last name followed by a comma, a single space, first name, a single space, and middle initial or name (if known). Examples: Shultz, Matthew Sr.

> Enter *Matthew Shultz Sr.* as the FAMILY
> HEAD NAME.

> **HINT:** To facilitate searching your database, it is very important that you follow the correct naming procedures.

23 Enter **ADDRESS** and **PHONE** information.

> Enter *1386 Quincy Lane, Allston, MA*
> *02134 703/464-0100* as address/phone
> information.

24 Tab through the yellow section of the *Families* form to the **NOTES** section. It may be necessary to click on the **ARROW** located below the yellow field in order to access the **NOTES** section of the form (see Figure 4-1). This field will store reminders that apply to the entire family. These reminders are in addition to the ones that are stored in each customer's record. Click in the **NOTES** data entry field. The white field turns blue when ready to accept information. Enter a short note in this field.

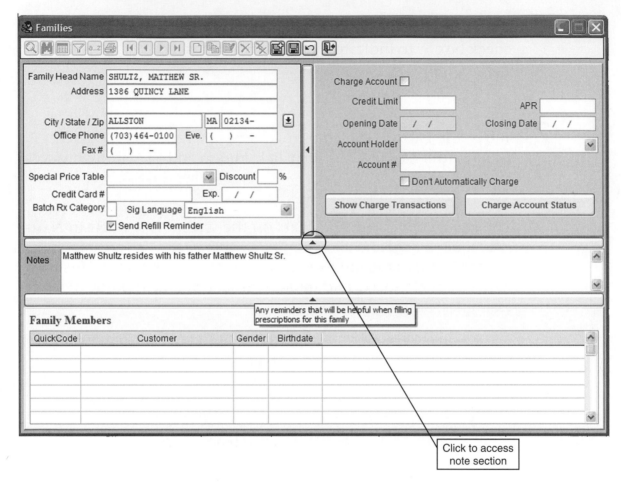

FIG **4-1**   Accessing note section.

25 Click on the **SAVE** icon located on the toolbar at the top right of the *Families* dialog box. Then click on the **CLOSE** icon located on the toolbar at the top right of the *Families* dialog box. The family head of household information has now been added to the database. The *Customers* dialog box is again active and ready for the form to be completed.

26 Click on the **ARROW** located to the right of the **LOCATION CODE** data entry field. Make the appropriate selection from the drop-down list.

Select *Home.*

27 Tab to the **Notes** field. In this field you can enter whatever information you want to store about the patient. The information will appear on the *Prescription Processing Screen* as a reminder when filling a prescription for this patient.

Enter *Matthew lives with his father.
Mother has visitation.*

28 The bottom half of the *Customers* form contains many tabs. Click on the **Allergies** tab.

29 Click on the **Add a New Record** icon located on the bottom right of the *Customers* form. An *Allergy Lookup* table pops up to access a list of allergies.

Select *No Known Allergies.*

30 Click on the **Other Drugs** tab. This grid contains information about other drugs that the patient is currently taking. These may be prescription drugs that were purchased from a different pharmacy, or they may be over-the-counter (OTC) drugs.

31 Click on the **Add a New Record** icon located on the bottom right of the *Customers* form. Press the **Enter** key to access a list of drugs. A *Drug Name Lookup* table pops up.

32 Look up the drug by typing the name of the drug in the **Name** dialog box. Click on the desired drug to select. Click on **OK**.

Select *Vitamin C 250 mg tablet
***chewable* for other drugs beginning on**
12/98.

33 Click on the **DISEASE PROFILE** tab. This grid contains a list of diseases the customer has been diagnosed for. The information contained in this grid is used to check for drug-disease contraindications each time a prescription is filled for the patient.

34 Click on the **ADD A NEW RECORD** icon located on the bottom right of the *Customers* form.

35 Press the **F2** key. A *Disease Lookup* table pops up entitled *CFDBDX*.

36 Look up the disease by typing the first few letters of the name of the disease. Click on the desired disease to select. Click on **OK**.

There is no disease state indicated for this customer. Click on *Cancel*.

36.1 Hit the ESC key to exit from the current EDIT mode completely.

36.2 Click on the EDIT icon to enter the editing mode for the next step.

37 Click on the **INSURANCE PLANS** tab. The insurance **PAYTYPE** is selected, therefore additional details such as *Insurance Plan, Cardholder ID, Group Number*, and so on must be provided. Click on the **NEW** icon located on the bottom right of the *Customers* form.

38 A **PICK LIST** appears on the table under the heading *Coverage Type*. Click on the **ARROW** to the right of the pick list and choose the appropriate coverage type from the drop-down list.

Choose *Primary*.

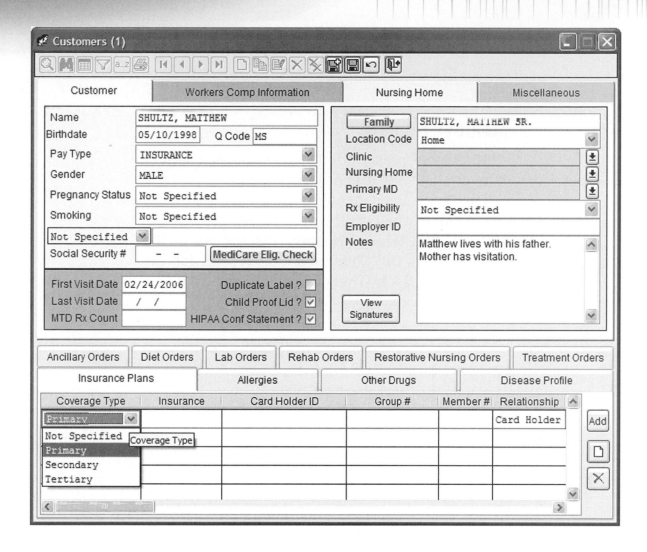

39 Press the **Tab** key and a new pick list appears entitled *Insurance*. Select the appropriate insurance plan. Click on **OK**.

Select *Advanced.*

40 Enter the *Cardholder ID, Group Number*, and *Member Number*.

Member Number

At the time of prescription drop-off, ask the patient if he or she is the primary card holder.

Primary is the card holder known as member 01 or 00. Input the correct card holder code in the computer as **MEMBER NUMBER**. The spouse of the cardholder is 02. Children are coded 03 for the oldest child, 04 for the middle child, and so on.

Advanced Insurance Co.

Primary Insured: Matthew Shultz
ID # 05877922130
Group# 70752
Bin# 004336
Rx ID# 1122541
Effective Date: 07/03/2006

41 Click on the **SAVE** icon located at the top right of the toolbar.

42 Print the screen by using the **PRINTSCRN** option on your keyboard: Press the **PRINTSCRN** key, open a blank Word document, **RIGHT CLICK** the blank Word document, and then select **PASTE**.

43 Click the **CLOSE** icon located at the top right of the toolbar.

Exercise

Enter the following customers into the database using the information provided.

> *MAMSI*
>
> **Primary Insured:** Ray Ruhl
> **ID #** FMK3332225521
> **Group #** FJT03
> **BIN #** 4000004
> **Rx ID #** 610052
> **Effective Date:** 12/01/2005
> **Electronic Processor:** MPN HCS

Patient and HOH: Ray Ruhl
DOB: 2/21/57
SSN: 472-97-4562
Allergies: PCN
170 Laurel Way
Herndon, VA 20170
703-481-5200
Requests easy-open caps
Other meds: albuterol inhaler, Singulair 10 mg
Disease State: seasonal allergies

> *PCS*
>
> Gamble, Robert   01
> **ID #** JK2233669875232
> **Group #** JS236
> **Rx BIN #** 610415
> **Electronic Processor:** 3211203827

Patient and HOH: Robert Gamble
DOB: 3/15/57
Allergies: PCN
1447 Woodbrook Court
Reston, VA 20194-1215
703-787-9000
Hospice patient
Requests easy-open lids
Disease State: CA
Other Medications: pain meds

PDS

Douglas, Doug   01
Douglas, Julie   02
ID # 7745LK236
Group # 525
Rx BIN: 4000004
Electronic Processor: HCS

Patient: Julie Douglas
HOH: Doug Douglas (same address as Julie)
DOB: 8/14/77
Allergies: codeine
Not pregnant
SSN: 333-56-9887
12124 Walnut Branch Road
Audubon, IA 50025
571-203-0000
Notes: Deliver prescriptions to home address before 5:00 PM

Antham

Cald, Timothy   01
Cald, Katherine   02
ID # 7521TIO2369
Group # N23
BIN: 610575
Electronic Processor: 00890000

PCS

Employer: Danish Home
Primary Insured: Cald, Katherine
ID # 4521212123
Rx Group # 4523
Rx BIN: 610415
Electronic Processor: 3211203827

Patient: Katherine Cald
HOH: Timothy Cald
DOB: 3/20/57
DL# I4569821
Allergies: cephalosporins
Insurance Plan: Anthem
11200 Longwood Grove
Elk Horn, IA 51531
703-464-1700

BCBSNJ

Primary Insured: Mang, Annette
ID # 78YT56
Rx Group # 23956
Rx BIN: 610014
Electronic Processor: HCS

Patient and HOH: Annette Mang
DOB: 1/21/57
SSN: 362-89-5663
Allergies: MSO_4
1490 Autumn Ridge Court
Reston, VA 20194-1215
703-834-0500
Other medications: alprazolam 1 mg, Seroquel 25 mg
Wants duplicate labels

Cigna

Primary Insured: Walks, Dana
ID # LMN236911236
Rx Group # PO1259
Rx BIN: 600428
Electronic Processor: 01060000

Patient and HOH: Dana Walks
DOB: 4/21/57
Allergies: PCN
1206 Weatherstone Court
Ralston, NE 68128
703-430-6300
Requests easy-open caps
Notes: Has not signed HIPAA
Other medications: Skelaxin 400 mg PRN, spironolactone 100 mg

Patient and HOH: Martin Marin
DOB: 5/17/50
Allergies: NKA
11324 Olde Tiverton Circle
Ralston, NE 68128
703-437-5000
Other medications: Aldactone 100 mg, Serevent Inhaler
Would like 2 labels
Would like easy-open caps
Work-related injury
Contact at work: Steve Fister—Manager
Bonds, Inc. @ 309 3rd St., Fister, NE 68110
Work phone: 402-698-2356

Making a Change to the Patient Profile

LAB OBJECTIVES

In this lab, you will:

- learn how to update the patient profiles
- review skills learned in Lab 4: Advanced Exercise—Adding a New Patient to the Database in order to change and update insurance information

Student Directions

Estimated completion time: 15 minutes

1. Read through the steps before performing the lab exercise on your computer.
2. After reading through the lab, perform the required steps to edit patient information.
3. Complete the exercise at the end of the lab.

Steps

1 Access the main screen of Visual SuperScript.

2 Click on the **CUSTOMERS** button located on the left side of the screen.

3 A dialog box entitled *Customers* will pop up.

4 Click on the **FIND** icon, which is located on the top left of the *Customers* dialog box toolbar.

5 A dialog box entitled *Customer Lookup* pops up. Enter the first letter of the customer's last name into the **NAME** data entry field. Click on the patient name to which information will be updated.

Find and select *John M. Smith.*

6 The selected customer name is highlighted in blue. Click on **EDIT** located at the bottom of the *Customer Lookup* dialog box.

7 A dialog box entitled *Customers* pops up. The *Customers* dialog box contains four tabbed forms. Click on the white tab entitled *Customer*.

8 Click on the **EDIT** icon 🖺 located in the middle of the *Customers* toolbar at the top of the dialog box.

9 The form is now ready to edit patient information. **TAB** to the desired data entry field and key in the appropriate changes.

Change John M. Smith's DOB to *02/22/1947*.

HINT: The active data entry field will be highlighted. Delete the existing information before adding the new information.

10 Click on the **SAVE** icon located on the toolbar at the top right of the *Customers* dialog box. Then click on the **CLOSE** icon located on the toolbar at the top right of the *Customers* dialog box. The edited information has now been added to the database.

11 Make note of the updated information in the *Customer Lookup* dialog box. Click on **OK** at the bottom of the *Customer Lookup* dialog box.

12 Print the screen by using the **PRINTSCRN** option on your keyboard: Press the **PRINTSCRN** key, open a blank Word document, **RIGHT CLICK** the blank Word document, and then select **PASTE**.

Exercise

Practice using the software data entry skills by entering the following patient information. Submit work when completed.

1. Change the following patient information:
Jada Sanchez's birthday is 08/30/1996
Margaret Pena's evening phone number is 555-639-5489

Scenario

Mr. Donald Peterson arrives at the pharmacy requesting a refill on his Clozaril 25 mg prescription. After viewing Mr. Peterson's prescription history, it is found that Mr. Peterson will need a new prescription from his physician. The Clozaril 25 mg prescription for Mr. Peterson that the pharmacy has on file has expired.

Mr. Peterson offers a new prescription for the medication when he is informed of the situation. "I'm sorry," Mr. Peterson explains, "I didn't know that you would need this new prescription." Mr. Peterson further explains, "Now that I think about it, maybe my insurance has changed since the last time I filled a prescription."

Task

Update Mr. Donald Peterson's insurance information.

Advanced Prescription Insurance

Primary Insured: Peterson, Donald
ID # 7459863
Rx Bin: 447225
Group ID: G56239
Coverage begins: 12/01/2006 – 12/01/2010

Note to Pharmacy: Electronic prescriptions are submitted to Advance PCS. PCS is the electronic biller.

Editing a Prescriber Form

LAB OBJECTIVES

In this lab, you will:

- learn how to make changes to the prescriber information form in the database. The DOCTOR/PRESCRIBER form may need to be updated from time to time. Each record or form in the doctor database contains several data elements or fields. Not all the fields are required when you add a new record to the database. However, information may be obtained at a later date, and the form will need to be edited in order to add the newly acquired information. It is relatively easy to make changes to the DOCTOR/PRESCRIBER form.

- be introduced to one of the many shortcuts available in the Visual SuperScript software program. You will find that the shortcut saves time when editing information in the database.

Student Directions

Estimated completion time: 15 minutes

1. Read through the steps before performing the lab exercise on your computer.
2. After reading through the lab, perform the required steps.
3. Complete the exercise at the end of the lab.

Steps

1 Access the main screen of Visual SuperScript.

2 Click on the **Doctors** button located on the left side of the screen.

3 A dialog box entitled *Doctors* will pop up.

4 Click on the **Find** icon located on the toolbar at the top of the dialog box. The *Find* dialog box appears.

5 The *Find* dialog box gives several choices for locating the prescriber's records. Key in the prescriber's last name in the **Name** data entry field. Click on **OK** at the bottom of the dialog box.

Key in *Dr. Robert Bosworth.*

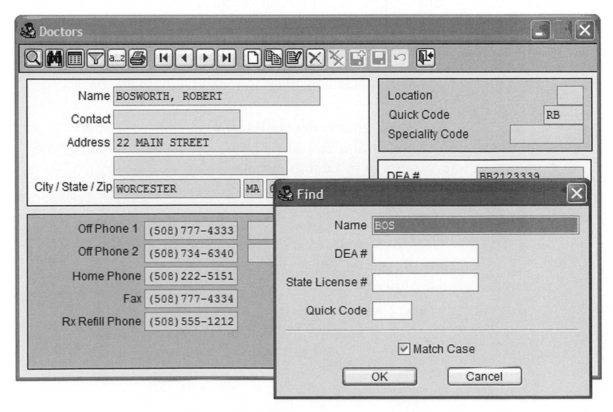

••••Shortcut Enter the first letter of the prescriber's last name into the Nᴀᴍᴇ data entry field. Click on **OK** at the bottom of the dialog box. A dialog box entitled *List* pops up. Scroll through the table in the *List* dialog box and select the desired prescriber by clicking on the prescriber's name. Click on **OK** located at the bottom of the *List* dialog box.

6 Click on the **Eᴅɪᴛ** icon located on the toolbar at the top of the form. The form is now ready for you to edit the prescriber information.

7 Tab through the form to reach the desired data entry field. Make appropriate changes to the form.

Office Phone 2 extension is *104*.

HINT: See Labs 1 and 2 for explanation of data entry fields on the **Dᴏᴄᴛᴏʀs** form.

8 Click on the **Sᴀᴠᴇ** icon located at the top right of the toolbar.

9 Print the screen by using the **PʀɪɴᴛSᴄʀɴ** option on your keyboard: Hit the **PʀɪɴᴛSᴄʀɴ** key, open a blank Word document, **Rɪɢʜᴛ Cʟɪᴄᴋ** the blank Word document, and then select **Pᴀsᴛᴇ**.

10 Return from the Word document to Visual SuperScript. Click the **Cʟᴏsᴇ** icon located at the top right of the toolbar.

Exercise

Scenario

Dr. Karen Davis is a prescribing physician in your area. She has recently married and changed her last name to a hyphenated name: Dr. Karen Davis-Bendfeldt. The managing pharmacist has asked you to update Dr. Davis-Bendfeldt's records.

Task

Following the steps from the *Editing a Prescriber Form* exercise, edit Dr. Karen Davis-Bendfeldt's information. Print or save the form and submit it for verification.

HINT: It is *not* necessary to delete the existing information before adding the new information. Simply key the new information into the highlighted data entry field.

Adding Insurance Plans to the Database

LAB OBJECTIVES

In this lab, you will:

- learn how to add a new insurance plan to the database
- key information regarding insurance billing procedures

Student Directions

Estimated completion time: 45 minutes

1. Read through the steps before performing the lab exercise on your computer.
2. After reading through the lab, perform the required steps listed in the lab.
3. Answer the questions at the end of the lab.
4. Complete the exercise at the end of the lab.

Pre Lab Information

The insurance plan name could be the same name of the insurance company. However, each insurance company generally offers different plans. Not only do these plans have different restrictions and different copay requirements, but they may also need to be submitted with different BIN and/or PROCESSOR CONTROL numbers. Therefore *it is best not to associate plan names with insurance company names*.

Similarly, there are Pharmacy Benefits Managers, such as ARGUS and DPS, that process claims on behalf of large numbers of insurance companies. It is best not to associate plan names with the names of these processors either.

Most often each insurance plan that requires a unique combination of BIN and PROCESSOR CONTROL numbers should have a separate name and a separate record.

Steps

1 Access the main screen of Visual SuperScript.

2 Click on the **INSURANCE PLANS** button located on the left side of the screen.

3 A dialog box appears entitled *Insurance Plans*. This *Insurance Plans* form is used to maintain a database of insurance plans that your customers subscribe to. The *Insurance Plans* form contains three tabs. Click on the **INSURANCE PLAN DATA** tab.

4 Click on the **NEW** icon located on the toolbar at the top of the *Insurance Plans* dialog box. The form is ready for data entry.

5 Enter the name of the insurance plan in the **PLAN NAME** data entry field.

Enter *Medco* as the plan name.

6 Tab to the **COMPANY** data entry field. Click on the **ARROW** to the right of the data entry field. A pick list appears. Scroll through the pick list and choose the desired insurance company name by clicking on the name.

Choose *United Healthcare* as the company name.

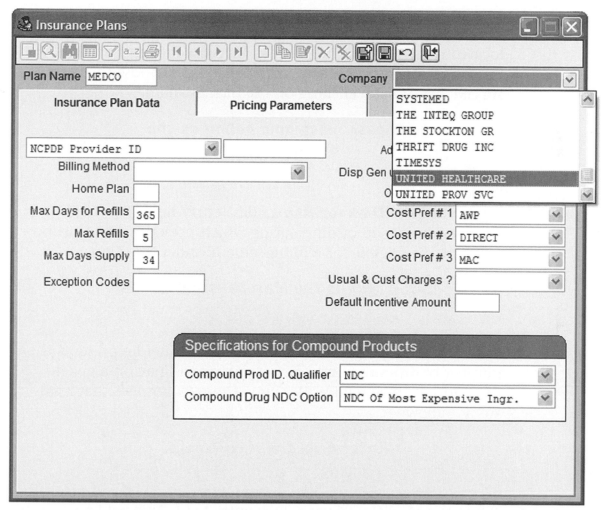

7 Tab to the next data entry field. This field is used to identify the pharmacy to the insurance company for billing purposes. Click on the **ARROW** located to the right of the data entry field. Scroll through the pick list and select the desired **IDENTIFICATION QUALIFIER** by clicking on the name.

Choose *National Council for Prescription Drug Programs (NCPDP)* as the identification qualifier.

8 Tab to the next data entry field. Enter the pharmacy identification number in the next data entry field. In most cases, the unique pharmacy identification number is the National Association Board of Pharmacy (NABP) number.

Enter *6503829* as the pharmacy ID.

9 Tab to the **BILLING METHOD** data entry field. Click on the **ARROW** located to the right of the **BILLING METHOD** data entry field. Several choices are available on the pick list. Choose the desired **BILLING METHOD** by clicking on the pick list name.

Choose *electronic billing* as the billing method.

10 Tab to the **MAX DAYS FOR REFILLS** data entry field. This field specifies the period of time during which prescriptions must be refilled to be eligible for reimbursement under this plan.

Enter *365* as the Max Days for Refills.

11 Tab to the **MAX REFILLS** data entry field. This field represents the number of times the insurance company will pay on a given prescription to be refilled. A value of zero (0) implies that refills are not allowed.

Enter *6* as the MAX REFILLS.

12 Tab to the **MAX DAYS SUPPLY** data entry field. This field represents a payer-imposed limit, if any, on the amount of a medication that may be dispensed at a time.

Enter *32* as the MAX DAYS SUPPLY.

13 Check the **ADD SALES TAX** check box ☑ if your state imposes a sales tax on medicines. The sales tax will then be billed to the insurance company.

HINT: To place a check mark in the check-off box, click in the box with your mouse button.

14 Check the **Disp Gen Unless DAW** box if the insurance company requires that generic drugs be dispensed unless the prescriber specifies "DAW" (dispense as written) on the prescription.

15 Check the **OTC Covered** box if over-the-counter (OTC) drugs are covered under this insurance plan.

OTC drugs are covered under this plan.

16 **Cost Prefs #1, #2**, and **#3** (cost preferences) are the three choices for calculating the ingredient cost of the drug. For each preference, the available choices are displayed in a pick list. Click the **Arrow** to the right of the data entry field to access the pick list. Select the three cost preferences. When pricing a prescription, Visual Superscript first attempts to calculate the ingredient cost based on **Cost Pref #1**. If **Cost Pref #1** is unavailable (as indicated by a zero in that field in the drug record), Visual Superscript then uses **Cost Pref #2**, and so on.

Enter *AWP* (average wholesale price) as Cost Pref #1.

Enter *MAC* (manufacturers' average cost) as Cost Pref #2.

Enter *Direct* as Cost Pref #3.

17 The **Usual & Cust Charges?** data entry field indicates whether or not the insurance company requires you to submit the usual and customary charge if the pharmacy price of the medication is lower than the price based on the ingredient-cost-plus-dispensing-fee formula specified by the insurance company. Click on the **Arrow** located to the right of the data entry field. Four options are provided on a drop-down list. Click on the desired drop-down list name.

Select *All Drugs* from the list.

18 Click on the yellow tab entitled *Pricing Parameters*. The *Pricing Parameters* form is active and ready for data entry.

19 Key in the desired markup factor in the **Brand Markup** data entry field. This is the factor by which the AWP (or MAC or direct cost) of the drug is multiplied to arrive at the ingredient cost of the drug for billing purposes. For example, a 10% markup should be entered as 1.1. A 100% markup should be entered as 2.00.

Enter *1* as the Brand Markup.

20 The *Brand* **Disp Fee** data entry field contains the dispensing fee allowed by the insurance company for brand-name drugs. The dispensing fee is added to the ingredient cost to arrive at the price of the drug. Key in the *Brand* **Disp Fee** allowed by the insurance company.

Enter *$3.50* as the Brand Disp Fee.

21 Key in the markup factor for brand-name OTC drugs in the *Brand* **Markup for OTC** data entry field.

Enter *1.25* as the Brand Markup for OTC.

22 Key in the amount of money (copay) to be paid by the customer for each brand-name prescription in the *Brand* **Copay** data entry field. The pharmacy collects the copay from the customer at the time the prescription is picked up from the pharmacy.

Enter 20 as the Brand Copay.

23 Check the **Is It Percent?** box if the figure entered in the copay field is to be treated as a percentage of the price rather than an absolute dollar amount. For example, if the price of the drug is $45.00 and there is an entry of 10 in the copay field and the **Is It Percent?** box is not checked, the copay computed by the system would be a $10.00 flat copay fee. However, if the **Is It Percent?** box is checked, the copay will be computed as $4.50 (10% of $45.00).

Leave the *Is It Percent?* box unchecked.

24 The *Brand* **Discount Copay** data entry field should reflect the same copay as the corresponding *Brand* copay field *unless* your pharmacy has decided to offer a lower copay amount than required by the insurance company. Key in the correct *Brand* **Discount Copay** and **Is It Percent?** information.

25 Key in the required information in the second column of the *Pricing Parameters* form. The second column is entitled *Generic*.

Generic Markup: 1

Generic Disp. Fee: $3.50

Generic Markup for OTC: 1

Generic Copay: $5

Generic Is It Percent? No

Generic Discount Copay: $5

Generic Is It Percent? No

26 Tab to the **Same Copay as Generics for Brand Drugs with No Gen** field. Usually, lower copays are required for generic drugs versus brand-name drugs as an incentive for patients to choose generic over brand-name drugs. Under some plans, the customer is allowed to pay the lower copay when a drug has no generics available. Check this box if the copays for brand-name and generic drugs are different and the insurance company allows the customer to pay the same copay as generics for brand-name drugs that have no generics available.

Check the Same Copay as Generics box.

27 Tab to the **Max Payment for an Rx** field. This field specifies the maximum amount the insurance company will pay for a single prescription.

There is no such limit—enter a large value such as 9999.

28 The **Perc. of Cost Diff. between Brand & Generics Paid** field specifies the *percentage* of the difference between the price of the brand-name and generic drugs that the insurance company requires the patient to pay if the patient chooses a brand-name drug over the generic. Enter the correct percentage difference in the **Perc. of Cost Diff. between Brand & Generics Paid** field.

Enter 80% (80.00) as the percentage of cost difference.

29 Click on the **Electronic Billing Options** tab. The *Electronic Billing Options* form is active and ready for data entry. The information contained in the *Electronic Billing Options* form determines to whom claims are sent for adjudication, as well as the format in which they are sent. Successful adjudication requires that all items must be entered as completely and accurately as possible.

30 The **EL. BILLER** (electronic biller) data entry field specifies the company to which the electronic claim is delivered initially. Click on the **COMBO-BOX DOWN ARROW** located to the right of the **EL. BILLER** data entry field. A dialog box entitled *Insurance Carrier* pops up. Select the appropriate company from the table by clicking on the company name. Then click on **OK** located at the bottom of the *Insurance Carrier* dialog box.

**Select *National Data Corp.* as the
insurance carrier.**

31 The **BIN** (biller identification number) identifies the party to whom the electronic biller (from step 29) needs to forward the claim. This field is required for all electronically transmitted plans. Most insurance companies will list the **BIN** on the insurance card issued to the customer. The **BIN** always consists of six numeric characters. Key in the correct **BIN**.

Enter *510455* as the BIN.

32 The **PROC. CTRL. #** (processing control number, or PCS) field is a required field for all electronically transmitted plans. The processing control number may also be referred to as the Carrier ID. Key in the appropriate Carrier ID.

Enter *HCS* as the PCS/Carrier ID.

33 Tab to the **REQUIRED MD ID** (required medical doctor/prescriber identification) data entry field. Click on the **ARROW** located to the right of the data entry field. Click on and select the appropriate identification number type that the insurance company uses to identify the prescriber. For successful adjudication, it is imperative that the appropriate identifier for each specific plan is selected.

Select *DEA#* as the identifier.

34 Click on the **Combo-box Down Arrow** located to the right of the **Default Other Coverage Code** data entry field. Click on the appropriate coverage code from the table in the *Default Other Coverage Code* dialog box. Click on **OK** located at the bottom of the dialog box.

Select *0–Not Specified* as the code.

35 Click on the **Combo-box Arrow** located to the right of the **Default Oth Cov Code for Secondary Billing** data entry field. Click on the appropriate coverage code from the table in the *Default Other Coverage Code* dialog box. Click on **OK** located at the bottom of the dialog box.

Select *0–Not Specified* as the code.

36 Click on the **Combo-box Arrow** located to the right of the **Default Rx Origin Code** data entry field. Indicate if the third-party payer (insurance company) requires prescriptions to be written (select *1—Written Prescription*) or if the third-party payer has no preference on the form or origin of the prescription (select *0—Not Specified*). After choosing the correct prescription origin code, click on **OK** located at the bottom of the *Rx Origin Code* dialog box.

Select *0–Not Specified* as the code.

37 Click on the **Combo-box Arrow** located on the right side of the **Default Rx Denial Override Code** data entry field. Select the correct denial override code from the table in the dialog box. Click on **OK** located on the bottom of the *Denial Override Code* dialog box.

Select *00–Not Specified* as the code.

38 Tab to the right side of the *Electronic Billing Options* form. Click on the **COMBO-BOX ARROW** located on the right side of the **DEFAULT RX ELIG CLAR. CODE** data entry field. Select the correct prescription eligibility clarification code from the table in the dialog box. Click on **OK** located on the bottom of the *Rx. Elig Clar Code* dialog box.

Select *0—Not Specified* as the code.

39 The check boxes located on the right side of the *Electronic Billing Options* form are optional fields. Completion of these fields may be required for some insurance plans. To ensure proper adjudication of your claims, it may be necessary to call the insurance help desk to find out which fields are required. Check the appropriate boxes.

Insurance Plans

Plan Name MEDCO   Company UNITED HEALTHCARE

| Insurance Plan Data | Pricing Parameters | Electronics Billing Options |

El. Biller NATIONAL DATA CORP

Bin # 510455

Proc. Ctrl. # HCS

Software Certification ID

Plan ID

Required MD ID DEA #

Default Other Coverage Code 0

Default Oth Cov Code for Secondary Billing 0

Default Rx Origin Code 0

Default Customer Location Code 00

Default Rx Denial Override Code 00

Default Rx Elig Clar. Code 0

Xmit Multiple Claims ☑

Other Coverage Code Required for Reversal ☐

Agg. Amt. for All Other Payers ☐

Agg. Amt. for Each Other Payer ☐

Don't Xmit Compound Segment ☐

Xmit Clinical Segment ☐

Don't Xmit Copay for Secondary Billing ☐

Copay Only on Secondary Billing ☐

Xmit HCPCS Code for Supply Items ☐

Xmit Deductible co-Insurance ☐

Xmit COB Seg for Copay Only ☐

Xmit COB if Primary Rejects ☐

NCPDP Version 3A

Customer Last Name ☐	Sales Tax ☐	Incentive Amount ☐
Customer First Name ☐	Service Level ☐	Dec Qty ☐
Card Holder Last Name ☐	Primary MD ID ☐	MD Last Name ☐
Card Holder First Name ☐	Clinic ID ☐	Employer Address ☐
Customer Address ☐	Diag Code ☐	Carrier ID ☐
Phone ☐	Unit Dose Ind ☐	Injury Date ☐
Home Plan Code ☐	Alt Prod Type ☐	Claim Ref ☐

40 Checking the **Xmit Multiple Claims** (transmit multiple claims) check box will allow for transmitting of multiple claims in a single transaction. If this check box is not checked, claims will be transmitted one at a time.

Check the Xmit Multiple Claims check box by clicking in the check box with your mouse.

41 Tab to the bottom gray area of the *Electronic Billing Options* form. The **NCPDP Version** field is required for all electronically submitted plans. The NCPDP field determines the format in which the information will be transmitted to the insurance company. Click on the **Combo-box Arrow** located to the right of the data entry field. Select the correct NCPDP version from the table in the dialog box. Click on **OK** located on the bottom of the *NCPDP Version* dialog box.

Select *version 3A*.

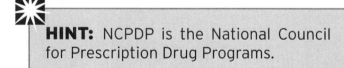

HINT: NCPDP is the National Council for Prescription Drug Programs.

42 Click on the **Save** icon located at the top of the *Insurance Plans* form. The insurance plan has now been added to the database.

43 Submit each tabbed area of the *Insurance Plans* form on completion.

Questions for Review

1 It is best to associate an insurance plan name with the name of the insurance company.

   a True

   b False

2 A pharmacy benefits manager is the entity that may process insurance claims for the insurance company.

   a True

   b False

3 The three tab names on the *Insurance Plans* form are

   _____, _____,

   and _____.

4 The IDENTIFICATION QUALIFIER is:

   a a coded number that identifies the insurance company.

   b used to identify the prescriber for third-party billing.

   c the same for every plan.

   d an optional data entry field.

5 BILLING METHOD choices include:

   a Electronic billing

   b Universal claim form

   c Fax

   d Both A and B

6 The MAX REFILLS data entry field represents:

a the maximum number of refills the pharmacy will allow the patient to have.

b the maximum number of refills the insurance plan will allow the patient to have.

c the number of times the insurance company will pay on a given prescription to be refilled.

d the maximum number of refills the prescriber will allow the patient to have.

7 Does your state impose a sales tax on prescription medications?

8 The copay for brand-name medications should always be marked as a percentage of the price of the medication.

a True

b False

9 An example of a third-party payer is the patient's insurance company.

a True

b False

10 The information contained in the *Electronic Billing Options* form:

a determines to whom claims are sent for adjudication.

b determines the format in which claims are sent.

c determines both A and B.

d determines patient copay amount, only.

11 The *Electronic Billing Options* form will be active only if the billing method choice is electronic billing.

a True

b False

12 The processing control number may also be referred to as the

_____ or the _____.

13 The BIN:

a identifies the party to whom the electronic biller needs to forward the claim.

b is a required field for all electronically transmitted plans.

c is a six-digit number on the customer's insurance card.

d all of the above.

14 NCPDP:

a named the official standard for pharmacy claims in the Health Insurance Portability and Accountability Act (HIPAA)

b National Council for Prescription Drug Programs

c provides pharmacies with a unique identifying number for interactions with federal agencies and third-party processors

d all of the above

Exercise

Scenario

The pharmacy manager has asked you to update the database by adding a new insurance plan. It is important to add the new plan by the end of the day in order to electronically submit a patient's prescription claim. Your manager provides you with a detailing of the pricing information:

Pharmacy ID: 6503829
Brand markup is 1.5 (Rx and OTC)
The pharmacy offers a discount only for generic drug copay: 1%

Task

Use the following insurance plan information, as well as the information that the managing pharmacist has provided, to add an insurance plan to the database. Select *Not Specified* for any insurance information that is not provided. Submit each tabbed area of the *Insurance Plans* form on completion.

Insurance Plan Information

Plan Name: SureWay
Plan Details: The maximum refills allowed is 12. The maximum days supply is 32. Refills are allowed for a maximum of 1 year. The pharmacy should always dispense generic medications unless otherwise indicated by the physician. If generic medication is not available, the customer will pay generic copay for brand-name medications. If generic medication is available, but the customer prefers brand-name medication, the customer must pay 90% of the price cost difference between brand and generic. All medications are subject to usual and customary charges. OTC drugs are not covered under this plan.

Company Name: SystemED
ID Qualifier: NCPDP—Format version 3A
Electronic Biller: Pro-Serv
BIN: 610053
Processor Control: 7Q 7700970
Cost Preference: AWP
Dispensing Fees: $3.00 brand/generic
Flat Copay: $10.00 Brand/$2.50 generic
Maximum Payment: None
Prescriber Qualifier: DEA number
Note: A code is required for claim reversal.

Quick Challenge

1 You have learned how to add a new insurance plan to the database. Can you add a new insurance company to the database?

a Right click the company name data entry field to access the add new insurance company dialog box.

b Key in name and address information.

c SAVE.

d Key in *All Protect* for insurance company. Use your school's address and phone information.

2 Can you add a new electronic biller to the database?

   a Right click the **EL. BILLER** data entry field to access the add new insurance billers dialog box.

   b Key in name and phone information.

   c SAVE.

   d Key in *BernieCheck* as the electronic biller. Create your own phone information.

3 Learn about Medicare prescription drug insurance in your state.

Adding Drugs to the Database

LAB OBJECTIVES

In this lab, you will:

- learn how to add medication inventory to the database

Student Directions

Estimated completion time: 45 minutes

1. Read through the steps before performing the lab exercise on your computer.
2. After reading through the lab, perform the required steps listed in the lab by using the Wellbutrin SR sample label.
3. Complete the scenario exercise at the end of the lab.

```
        Wellbutrin SR
          bupropion
         150 mg tablet

      NDC 58016-0599-90

   Southwood Pharmaceuticals


   Lot # B203442
   Exp. 12/2010
```

Steps

Refer to the drug label above to complete the following steps.

1 Access the main screen of Visual SuperScript.

2 Click on the **Drug** button located on the left side of the screen.

3 A dialog box appears entitled *Drugs*. This *Drugs* form is used to maintain a database of drugs that are dispensed in the pharmacy. The *Drugs* form contains three tabs. Click on the **Drug and Packaging** tab.

4 Click on the **New** icon located on the toolbar at the top to the *Drugs* dialog box. The form is ready for data entry.

5 **Drug Brand Name** is a required field. Enter the brand name of the drug that is to be added to the database.

6 The *All Drugs Lookup* dialog box pops up after entering the name of the drug. Scroll through the table of drugs and click on the correct drug that is to be added to the database. After selecting the correct drug, click on **OK** located on the bottom of the *All Drugs Lookup* dialog box. The drug name is automatically entered in the **Label Name** field.

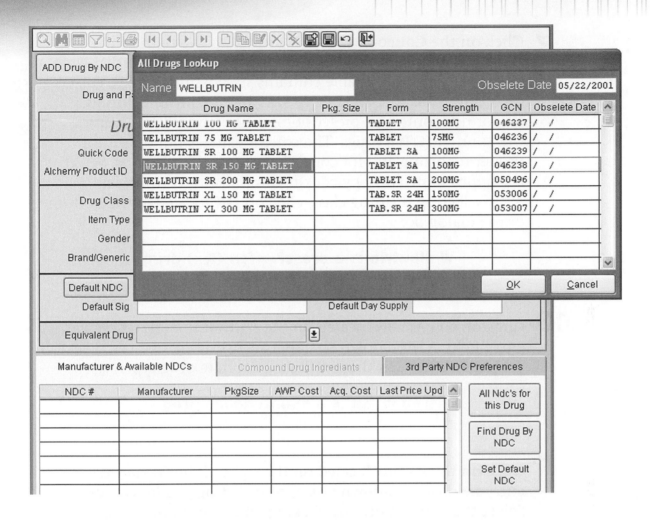

7 Tab to the **Quick Codes** data entry field. **Quick Codes** allow you to expedite the search for drugs when filling prescriptions. Enter the first few characters of the name of the drug in the **Quick Codes** data entry field.

8 The **Alchemy Product ID** field is automatically completed with the selection of the drug. It is important that the entry in this field is completed because this code produces all warning and counseling messages for the drug.

9 Click on the **COMBO-BOX ARROW** located to the right of the **DRUG CLASS** data entry field. A dialog box appears entitled *Drug Class*. The dialog box table contains six possible entries: *C2, C3, C4, C5* for Class or Schedule 2, 3, 4, and 5 controlled drugs; *RX* for noncontrolled prescription drugs; and *OT* for over-the-counter (OTC) drugs. The correct value is important for proper reporting and for correctly pricing prescriptions. Select the appropriate entry by clicking on the correct drug class. After selecting the drug class, click on **OK** located at the bottom of the dialog box.

Wellbutrin is a *prescription* (Rx) drug.

10 Click on the **ARROW** located on the right of the **ITEM TYPE** data entry field. A drop-down box appears listing six choices. Select the correct entry by clicking on the appropriate drug type.

Wellbutrin is a *maintenance* drug.

11 Click on the **ARROW** located on the right of the **GENDER** data entry field. A drop-down box appears listing gender choices. Select the correct entry by clicking on the appropriate gender description.

Select *Both* for Wellbutrin.

12 Click on the **ARROW** located on the right of the **BRAND/GENERIC** data entry field. Correctly identifying a drug as brand or generic is very important for third-party billing. For example, if a prescription is to be filled for a brand-name drug, the system can prompt a DAW code. Correct entry in this field is also important for pricing if the pharmacy has special tables for pricing generics. Select the correct entry by clicking on either brand or generic.

Wellbutrin is *Brand*.

13 Tab to the **Default Sig** data entry field. Certain drugs are frequently prescribed with the same instructions for use. Entering the appropriate instructions in this field can save time when filling a prescription.

> **Enter *T1TPOBID* as the sig code for "Take one tablet by mouth two times daily" for Wellbutrin instructions.**

14 Click on the **Combo-box Arrow** located to the right of the **Equivalent Drug** data entry field. A dialog box appears entitled *Eq. Drug Choices for...*A list of equivalent drugs is provided. For example, the name of a generic drug equivalent is provided for any brand-name drugs, and the name of a brand-name drug equivalent is provided for any generic drugs. Select the correct entry by clicking on the correct drug choice. Click on **OK** located at the bottom of the dialog box.

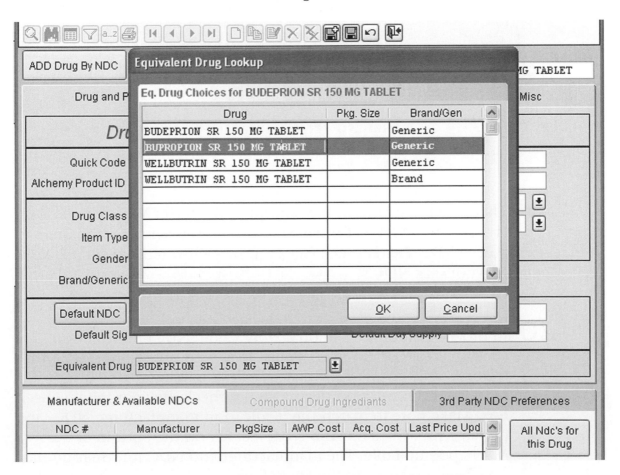

15 Tab to the right side of the form entitled Packaging. The **Form**, **Strength**, **Drug Unit**, and **Units** fields have automatically been updated to coincide with the selected medication.

16 Tab to the **Max Dose** data entry field. Key in the maximum daily dose advised for this particular medication.

**Enter 2 as the maximum dose
for Wellbutrin.**

17 Tab to the **Default Quantity** data entry field. Certain drugs are frequently prescribed with the same quantity instructions. Key in the desired quantity to be dispensed in the prescription for this particular medication.

**Enter 60 as the Default Quantity
for Wellbutrin.**

18 Tab to the **Default Day Supply** data entry field and key in the desired quantity.

**Enter 30 for Default Day Supply
for Wellbutrin.**

19 There are three tabs on the bottom of the form: **Manufacturer's & Available NDC's**, **Compounding Drug Ingredients**, and **3rd Party NDC Preferences**. Click on the yellow tab: **Manufacturer's & Available NDC's**.

20 In order to input the National Drug Code (NDC) information, click on **All NDC's for this drug** located on the right side of the form. A table pops up entitled *Add NDC's*. Using the medication label from the stock bottle as a guide, check the appropriate check box. Make note to match the medication manufacturer, NDC, and package size. Click on **Add NDC** located on the bottom of the *Add NDC's* pop-up table. The manufacturer and NDC information has now been updated on the *Drugs* form.

21 Make note that the NDC number, Manufacturer, Package Size, AWP Cost, Acquisition Cost, and Last Price Update have automatically been added to the table at the bottom of the *Drugs* form.

> **Click on the NDC number that has just been added to the table. Click on SET DEFAULT NDC located at the bottom of the form. Click on OK in the *Confirmation* dialog box. The NDC number has automatically been entered in the DEFAULT NDC data field under the *Drug* and *Packaging* tab.**

22 Click on the NDC number that has just been added to the *Drugs* form table. This NDC number will match the NDC number on the stock medication label. Click on the **EDIT** icon located on the bottom of the *Drugs* form. The Drug NDC dialog box appears. This dialog box allows for additional data entry.

23 Tab to the **LOT#** data entry field on the right side of the dialog box. Key in the medication lot number according to the stock bottle label.

24 Tab to the **EXPIRY DATE** data entry field. Key in the correct medication expiration date according to the stock bottle label. Click on **SAVE** at the bottom of the dialog box.

HINT: The **LOT #** and **EXPIRY DATE** will most likely change each time you receive new stock of the drug. To ensure that the entries in this field are current, you must update these values each time you begin to use the newly arrived stock.

25 Click on the yellow **PRICING AND STOCK** tab located at the top of the form. Click on the **EDIT** icon at the top of the form.

26 The **PRICE TABLE** is a required field that links each drug to a pricing formula for the purpose of calculating the usual and customary price of the drug. Click on the **ARROW** located to the right of the **PRICE TABLE** data entry field. Select the appropriate entry by clicking on the correct price table.

> **HINT:** BRN: brand-name drug
> GEN: generic drug
> OTC: over-the-counter drug

27 Tab to the area of the form entitled *General*. Key in the **MINIMUM STOCK** value that the pharmacy wishes to maintain for the new medication that is being added to the database.

**Enter *200* for minimum stock
of Wellbutrin.**

28 In the **REORDER QTY.** (reorder quantity) data entry field, key in the quantity of medication that the pharmacy will reorder when the stock is at its minimum.

**Enter *100* for reorder quantity
for Wellbutrin.**

29 The **VERIFIED STOCK** field is the total amount of drug that is on the shelf. This is the current amount of drug that is on the shelf plus the amount of drug that is being added to the pharmacy shelf. This amount could be tablets, capsules, or liquid form (milliliters). Key in the actual amount or quantity of medication that is on the pharmacy shelf in the **VERIFIED STOCK** data entry field.

> **Three stock bottles of Wellbutrin will be added to the pharmacy shelf. Each bottle contains 90 tablets. Therefore key in *270* in the Verified Stock data entry field.**

30 The **VERIFIED STOCK DATE** is the date that the new drug is being added to the pharmacy shelf and the date that physical inventory has been performed. Key in the correct date.

31 Tab to the **DAYS TO EXPIRE** data entry field. The value entered in this field is used to determine the expiration date that will be printed on prescription labels. The default value for this field is 1 year. Some drugs, such as reconstituted antibiotics, have a 10-day shelf life, a much shorter shelf life than 1 year. Make sure that you change this value appropriately. Key in the correct number of days.

32 Click on the **WELFARE & MISC** tab located at the top of the form.

33 Check the **TRIPLICATE SERIAL # REQD** check box to tag individual drugs for control drug reporting.

> **Wellbutrin is not a controlled drug. Do *not* check this check box.**

34 Check the **Prior Auth Required** check box if your state Medicaid department requires prior authorization to fill prescriptions for this drug. Visual Superscript will then prompt you for prior authorization whenever you fill a prescription for a Medicaid-covered patient for this drug.

35 Click on the **Save** icon located at the top of the *Drugs* form. The new drug has now been added to the pharmacy's working drug file.

36 Submit all tabbed areas of the form. Print the screen by using the **PrintScrn** option on your keyboard: key **PrintScrn**, open a blank Word document, **Right Click** the blank Word document, and then select **Paste**.

37 Click on the **Close** icon located at the top of the *Drugs* form.

Exercise

Scenario

Dr. Yard and Dr. R. Sill are the chief prescribers in your area. Typically these two physicians prescribe Viagra to treat symptoms associated with male impotence. Your pharmacy is well stocked with Viagra to meet the needs of patients who may be prescribed this medication by Dr. Yard or Dr. R. Sill.

Dr. M. Wickland has recently transferred to your area and set up practice at the neighborhood clinic. It has come to the managing pharmacist's attention that Dr. M. Wickland prescribes Levitra to treat symptoms associated with erectile dysfunction/male impotence. In the past, your pharmacy has not stocked Levitra, because there was not a demand for this medication in your area. It is now necessary to order Levitra from your pharmacy wholesaler.

Task

A shipment of Levitra (3 bottles) has arrived this morning in the pharmacy order. You have been assigned the responsibility of entering the new drug, Levitra, into your pharmacy database. On completion of the exercise, submit the form for verification.

```
┌─────────────────────────────────────┐
│           Physicians TC             │
│                                     │
│              Levitra                │
│       Vardenafil Hydrochloride      │
│            20mg Tablet              │
│                #4                   │
│                                     │
│                                     │
│   54868-4967-01                    │
│   Lot #1568                        │
│   12/2015                          │
│                                     │
└─────────────────────────────────────┘
```

Sig: T1TPO 1 hour before activity as the sig code for Take one tablet by mouth 1 hour before activity
Class: impotence agent/phosphodiesterase inhibitor
Default Days Supply: 1; quantity: 4; dose: 1
Reorder Quantity: 20
Pharmacy Minimum Stock: 30 tablets

Adding a Drug to the Database by NDC Number

LAB OBJECTIVES

In this lab, you will:

- build on skills learned in Lab 8: Adding Drugs to the Database by learning an alternative way to add new drugs to the database. This lab instructs on how to add a new drug to the database by National Drug Code (NDC) number.

Student Directions

Estimated completion time: 30 minutes

1. Read through the steps before performing the lab exercise on your computer.
2. After reading through the lab, perform the required steps to enter patient information.
3. Complete the exercise at the end of the lab.

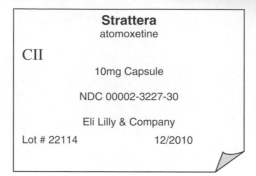

Strattera
atomoxetine

CII

10mg Capsule

NDC 00002-3227-30

Eli Lilly & Company

Lot # 22114   12/2010

Steps

Use the drug label above to complete the following steps.

1 Access the main screen of Visual SuperScript.

2 Click on the **Drug** icon located on the left side of the screen.

3 A dialog box appears entitled *Drugs*. This *Drugs* form is used to maintain a database of drugs that are dispensed in the pharmacy. Click on **Add Drugs by NDC** located at the top left side of the form.

4 A dialog box entitled *Add Drug by NDC* appears. Key in the NDC number as it appears on the stock bottle label. Select the appropriate entry by clicking on the correct NDC number. Click on **Add Drug** located at the bottom of the dialog box.

5 The *Drugs* form has now been updated with the new medication. Click on the **Edit** icon located on the bottom of the form.

6 The *Drug NDC* dialog box appears. Tab to the **Lot #** data entry field on the right side of the dialog box.

**Key in the drug lot number according to
the stock bottle label.**

7 Tab to the **Expiry Date** (expiration date) data entry field.

**Key in the drug expiration date
according to the stock bottle label.**

8 Click on the **Save** button at the bottom of the *Drug NDC* dialog box.

9 Click on the **Edit** icon located at the top of the *Drugs* form.

10 Tab to the **Quick Codes** data entry field. **Quick Codes** allow you to expedite the search for drugs when filling prescriptions.

**Enter the first few characters of the
name of the drug in the Quick Codes data
entry field.**

11 The **Alchemy Product ID** field is automatically completed with the selection of the drug. It is important that the entry in this field is completed because this code produces all warning and counseling messages for the drug.

12 Many data entry fields are automatically completed with the selection of the drug. The **Drug Class**, **Item Type**, **Gender**, and **Brand/Generic** fields have been updated to coincide with the drug selection. Tab to the **Default Sig** data entry field. Certain drugs are frequently prescribed with the same instructions for use. Entering the appropriate instructions in this field can save time when filling a prescription.

**Enter the sig abbreviation *T 1 T PO QD*
for "Take one tablet by mouth once
daily" for Strattera instructions.**

13 Tab to the **MAX DOSE** data entry field. Key in the maximum daily dose advised for this particular medication.

> **Enter *1* as the maximum dose for
> Strattera.**

14 Tab to the **DEFAULT QUANTITY** data entry field. Certain drugs are frequently prescribed with the same quantity instructions. Key in the desired quantity to be dispensed in the prescription for this particular medication.

> **Enter *30* as the default quantity
> for Strattera.**

15 Tab to the **DEFAULT DAY SUPPLY** data entry field and key in the desired quantity.

> **Enter *30*.**

16 Click on the yellow **PRICING AND STOCK** tab located at the top of the form.

17 The **PRICE TABLE** is a required field that links each drug to a pricing formula for the purpose of calculating the usual and customary price of the drug. The correct **PRICE TABLE** has automatically been added with the selection of the drug.

18 Tab to the area of the form entitled *General*. Key in the **MINIMUM STOCK** value that the pharmacy wishes to maintain for the new medication that is being added to the database.

> **Enter *90* for minimum stock of Strattera.**

19 In the **REORDER QTY.** (reorder quantity) data entry field, key in the quantity of medication that the pharmacy will reorder when the stock is at its minimum.

> **Enter *60* for reorder quantity for Strattera.**

20 The **VERIFIED STOCK** field is the amount of drug that is being added to the pharmacy shelf. This amount could be tablets, capsules, or liquid form (milliliters). Key in the actual amount or quantity of medication that will be added to the pharmacy shelf in the **VERIFIED STOCK** data entry field.

> **Five stock bottles of Strattera will be added to the pharmacy shelf. Each bottle contains 30 tablets. Therefore key in *150* in the verified stock data entry field.**

21 **STOCK VERIFICATION DATE** is the date that the new drug is being added to the pharmacy shelf.

> **Key in the correct date.**

22 Click on the **WELFARE & MISC** tab located at the top of the form.

23 Check the **TRIPLICATE SERIAL # REQD** check box to tag individual drugs for control drug reporting.

24 Check the **PRIOR AUTH REQUIRED** check box if your state Medicaid department requires prior authorization to fill prescriptions for this drug. Visual SuperScript will then prompt you for prior authorization whenever you fill a prescription for a Medicaid-covered patient for this drug.

25   Click on the **SAVE** icon located at the top of the *Drugs* form. The new drug has now been added to the pharmacy's working drug file.

26   Click on the **CLOSE** icon located at the top of the *Drugs* form.

Exercise

Using your data entry skills, add the following drugs to the pharmacy inventory. On completion of the exercise, submit the forms for verification.

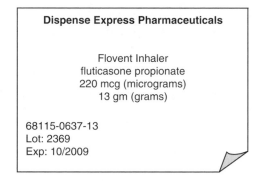

Sig abbreviation code:
U2S EN QD sig code for: Use two sprays in each nostril once daily.
Note: Five inhalers were received in the order. Four inhalers are currently on the shelf.

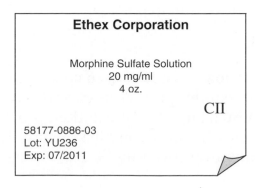

Sig abbreviation code:
T1DR PO PC and HS PRN sig code for: Take one teaspoonful by mouth after meals and at bedtime as needed.
Note: One bottle received in order. Two bottles currently on the shelf.

Quick Challenge

1 You have learned how to add drugs to the software database. In reading the steps in Labs 8 and 9, you have come to understand that the pharmacy will order and update stock on a regular basis. Can you complete an electronic purchase order used to order medication stock for the pharmacy?

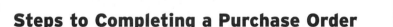

Steps to Completing a Purchase Order

a. Click on **INVENTORY** on the menu toolbar.
b. Click on **EXPORT DRUG STOCK ORDER**.
c. Press the **F2** key to access a list of pharmacy-approved **VENDORS**.
d. Double-click on the desired vendor.
e. Place a check mark in the check box of the drugs that need to be on the order.
f. Click on **ADD** and then click on the **F2** key to add a new drug to the purchase order.
g. **PREVIEW** the *Purchase Order*.
h. Click on **EXPORT** to electronically submit the order to the vendor.

2 Order the following stock from XYZ Drugs, Inc. Print the purchase order and submit for verification.

- Reorder Quantity: 56-Prempro 0.625/2.5 mg tab #00046-0875-6
- Reorder Quantity: 200-Synthroid 125 mcg #00048-1130-03
- Reorder Quantity: 90-Nexium 20 mg capsule #00186-5020-31
- 1-Urea Powder

REPORTS

Customer History Report

LAB OBJECTIVES

In this lab, you will:

- learn how to create a pharmacy business report that details the patient/customer prescription history

Student Directions

Estimated completion time: 15 minutes

1. Read through the steps before performing the lab exercise on your computer.
2. After reading through the lab, perform the required steps to generate a customer history report.
3. Complete the exercise at the end of the lab.

Steps

1 Access the main screen of Visual SuperScript.

2 Click on **REPORTS** from the menu toolbar located at the top of the screen.

3 Select **CUSTOMER REPORTS** from the drop-down menu. Then select **CUSTOMER HISTORY** from the expanded menu.

4 The *Customer History* dialog box appears. Notice that the insertion point is in the first data entry field, **DATE FROM**. Key in the date that the *Customer History Report* should start. It is not necessary to delete the default date that appears in the data entry field. The date that is keyed in will replace the existing default date.

Key in *01/20/2005*.

5 Key in the date that the *Customer History Report* should end in the **To** data entry field.

Key in *12/31/2005*.

6 The **SHOW** field will designate if the report should be generated to show the **COPAY** amount for the medications or the actual **PRICE** of the medications. **CLICK** on the appropriate choice.

Select *Copay*.

7 The **FORMAT** field will designate if the report should be generated in an **INSURANCE** format or a **NHOME** (nursing home) format. Select **INSURANCE** format unless the patient is a resident of a nursing home. Click on the appropriate choice.

Select *Insurance.*

8 Select the **NEW PAGE FOR EACH CUSTOMER** field if individual pages are desired.

9 The **FOR** data field offers several different choices in generating the *Customer History Report.* Select one of the five choices in which the *Customer History Report* will be generated. Click on the appropriate choice.

Select *Individual* Customer.

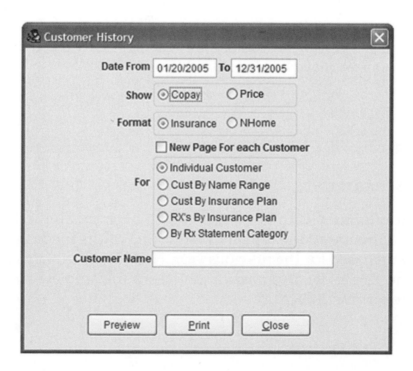

10 The last **NAME** data entry field will ask for the customer name or the name of the insurance plan. The required information depends on the selection made in step 9. Key in the appropriate information.

Key in *Posner, Rose* (you may use a shortcut and key in the patient's initials followed by F2 for customer lookup).

11 Click on **PREVIEW** located the bottom of the *Customer History* dialog box. The selected *Customer History Report* will open and appear on the screen.

12 Click on the **PRINT REPORT** icon 🖨 located at the top right of the *Report Designer* toolbar.

13 Click on the **CLOSE PREVIEW** icon 🚪 located at the top right of the *Report Designer* toolbar. The report is closed out and the *Customer History* dialog box returns.

Exercise

Scenario

It is January 10th of the new year. Mr. Harry Zinn calls your pharmacy asking for a detailed listing of the medications that he purchased for the previous year. Harry Zinn explains that he needs the detailed medication record to complete his income tax report for 2005.

Task

Following the steps from the *Reporting Customer History* exercise, compile a detailed listing of Mr. Harry Zinn's medications for the year 2005. Print the report and submit it for verification.

1. What was the total out-of-pocket expense that Mr. Zinn paid to your pharmacy in 2005 for prescription medication?
2. How many tablets did Mr. Zinn receive on his 04/06/2005 prescription for Celebrex?

Control Drug Report

In this lab, you will:

- learn how to create a pharmacy business report that details the inventory and dispensing activity of controlled medications in the pharmacy

Student Directions

Estimated completion time: 15 minutes

1. Read through the steps before performing the lab exercise on your computer.
2. After reading through the lab, perform the required steps to generate a control drug report.
3. Complete the exercise at the end of the lab.

Steps

1 Access the main screen of Visual SuperScript.

2 Click on **REPORTS** from the menu toolbar located at the top of the screen.

3 Select **DRUG REPORTS** from the drop-down menu. Then select **CONTROL DRUG REPORT** from the expanded menu.

4 The *Control Drug Report* dialog box appears. Notice that the insertion point is in the first data entry field, **DATE FROM**. Key in the date that the *Control Drug Report* should start. It is not necessary to delete the default date that appears in the data entry field. The date that is keyed in will replace the existing default date.

Key in *01/01/2005.*

5 Key in the date that the *Control Drug Report* should end in the **To** data entry field.

Key in *03/01/2005.*

6 The **DRUG SELECTION** field will designate if the report will generate a list of Class/Schedule II drugs only: **C2 ONLY;** Class/Schedule III through Class/Schedule V: **C3–C5** drugs; or **ALL (C2–C5)** drugs. Click on the appropriate choice.

Select *All (C2-C5).*

7 The **Sort By** field will designate in what order the report should be arranged. Indicate how the report should be arranged: **Fill Date**, **Drug Name**, or **Customer**. Click on the appropriate choice.

Select *Drug Name*.

8 Click on **Preview** located at the bottom of the *Control Drug Report* dialog box. The selected *Control Drug Report* will open and appear on the screen.

9 Click on the **Print Report** icon located at the top right of the *Report Designer* toolbar.

10 Click on the **Close Preview** icon located at the top right of the *Report Designer* toolbar. The report is closed out and the *Control Drug Report* dialog box returns.

Exercise

Scenario

The managing pharmacist is reconciling the CII logbook. There is a discrepancy in methylphenidate 5 mg. The CII logbook indicates that the pharmacy should have 140 tablets in stock. However, the physical count of methylphenidate 5 mg is 160 tablets. The managing pharmacist has asked for your help in finding out where the discrepancy between the CII logbook and the actual medication in stock occurred.

Task

Following the steps from the *Drug Reports: Control Drug Report* exercise, compile a detailed listing of dispensed methylphenidate 5 mg from 01/01/2005 to 03/01/2005. Print the report and submit it for verification.

1. What is the number of methylphenidate 5 mg tablets that were dispensed from the pharmacy between 01/08/2005 and 02/13/2005?

2. What are the three *Control Drug Report* sort choices?

Quick Challenge

1 You are becoming more and more familiar with the Visual SuperScript software system. Can you find the main menu option that will print a list of top-selling drugs?

a Print a *Top-Selling Drug Report* listing the 10 top-selling drugs by AWP from 01/01/2005 through 06/30/2005. Submit the report for verification.

b What is the name of the top-selling or top-performing drugs for this time period?

Activity Summary Report

LAB OBJECTIVES

In this lab, you will:

- learn how to create and format a pharmacy business report that details the dispensing activity for the pharmacy

Student Directions

Estimated completion time: 15 minutes

1. Read through the steps before performing the lab exercise on your computer.
2. After reading through the lab, perform the required steps to generate an activity summary report.
3. Complete the exercise at the end of the lab.

Steps

1 Access the main screen of Visual SuperScript.

2 Click on **REPORTS** from the menu toolbar located at the top of the screen.

3 Select **ACTIVITY SUMMARY** from the drop-down menu.

4 The *Summary* dialog box appears. There are four choices on how the *Prescription Activity Summary Report* can be generated: **DAILY**, **MONTHLY**, **YEARLY**, or **DATE RANGE**. Click on the appropriate choice. Key in the desired date.

Select *Monthly*. Key in *05/2005*.

5 The **COST BY** field will designate if the report should be generated to show the **AWP** for medications dispensed during the selected date(s) or the **ACQ** (acquisition price) of the medications. Click on the appropriate choice.

Select *AWP*.

6 Click on **SUMMARY** located the bottom of the *Summary* dialog box. The selected *Prescription Activity Summary Report* will open and appear on the screen.

7 Click on the **Print Report** icon located at the top right of the *Report Designer* toolbar.

8 Click on the **Close Preview** icon located at the top right of *the Report Designer* toolbar. The report is closed out and the *Summary* dialog box returns.

9 Click on **Details** located at the bottom of the *Summary* dialog box.

10 A *Summary Details Report* for the selected date(s) appears on the screen. This report gives a more detailed view of the prescription activity for the selected timeframe.

11 Click on the **Print Report** icon located at the top right of the *Report Designer* toolbar.

12 Click on the **Close Preview** icon located at the top right of the *Report Designer* toolbar. The report is closed out and the *Summary* dialog box returns.

Exercise

Print a monthly *Prescription Activity Summary Report* for 11/2005. Submit the report for verification.

1. How many new prescriptions did the pharmacy fill in 11/2005?
2. What are the names of the medications filled from the pharmacy in 11/2005?
3. What was the total revenue for 11/2005?

Daily Prescription Log Report

LAB OBJECTIVES

In this lab, you will:

- learn how to create a report that summarizes the pharmacy dispensing records. Many states require a hard copy of all electronic records to be kept on file at the pharmacy.

Student Directions

Estimated completion time: 25 minutes

1. Read through the steps before performing the lab exercise on your computer.
2. After reading through the lab, perform the required steps to generate a daily prescription log report.
3. Complete the exercise at the end of the lab.

Steps

1 Access the main screen of Visual SuperScript.

2 Click on **REPORTS** from the menu toolbar located at the top of the screen.

3 Select **DAILY PRESCRIPTION LOG** from the drop-down menu. Then select **DAILY RX LOG** from the expanded menu.

> **HINT:** Select an item by left-clicking on the item with your mouse.

4 The *Daily Rx Log* dialog box appears. The **SELECT** section of the dialog box offers three choices on information that will be included in the *Daily Prescription Log Report:* **ALL PRESCRIPTIONS, NEW PRESCRIPTIONS ONLY,** or **REFILLS ONLY.** Click on the appropriate choice.

Select *All Prescriptions.*

5 Key in the desired date range in the **INCLUDE RECORDS FROM** field.

Key in *11/01/2005* to *12/31/2005.*

6 The **AGGREGATION TYPE** field allows for formatting choices in the report. Choose **SEPARATE EACH DAY** if the report should have prescription information from each date on a separate page. Choose **COMBINED FOR PERIOD** if the report should have prescription information flow from one page to another, regardless of the date. Click on the appropriate choice.

Choose *Separate Each Day.*

7 Choose the amount of information that should be included on the *Daily Prescription Log* report in the **Detail Level** section of the *Daily Rx Log* dialog box. **Detail Level One** is the basic report providing prescription information. **Detail Level Two** provides the patient address in addition to the basic information. **Detail Level Three** provides patient and prescriber address, as well as the NDC number of the dispensed medication in addition to the basic information. Click on the appropriate choice.

Choose *Detail Level Three.*

8 Click on the **Show Cost Using** check box. Designate if the report should be generated to show the **AWP** medication cost for prescriptions dispensed during the selected date(s) or the **Acquisition** cost of the medications dispensed. Click on the appropriate choice.

Select *AWP.*

9 The **Sort by Section** of the dialog box allows four different formats in sorting or arranging the *Daily Prescription Log* report: **Fill Date**, **Drug Class**, **Rx #**, or **Pay Type**. Click on the appropriate choice.

Choose *Fill Date.*

10 Click on **Preview** located on the bottom of the *Daily Rx Log* dialog box. The selected *Daily Prescription Log Report* will open and appear on the screen.

11 Click on the **Print Report** icon located at the top right of the *Report Designer* toolbar. Be sure to print only the pages necessary for this report.

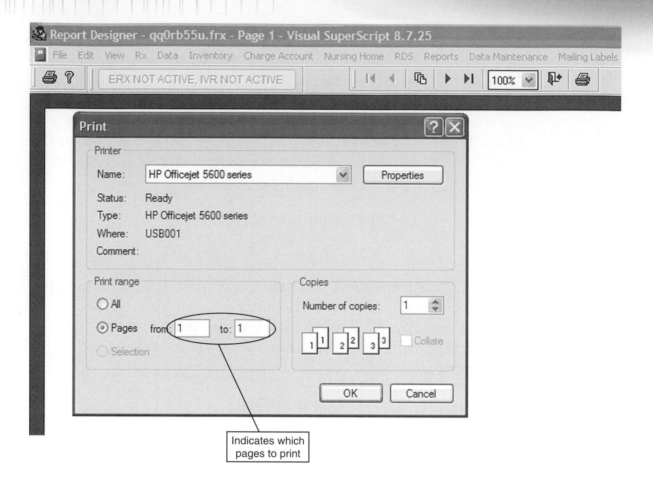

Indicates which
pages to print

12 Click on the **Close Preview** icon located at the top right of the *Report Designer* toolbar. The report is closed out and the *Daily Rx Log* dialog box returns.

13 Click on **Close** located at the bottom of the *Daily Rx Log* dialog box.

Exercise

Scenario

The pharmacy manager has asked you to compile a report that summarizes the prescriptions dispensed for last month (May 2005). The manager would like the report arranged by third-party payers. The report should include the NDC number of the dispensed drug. The manager has also told you that the report will be filed as a hard-copy record or backup record in case of system failure.

Task

Following the steps presented in this lab, compile a *Daily Prescription Log Report* that will meet the pharmacy manager's needs. Print the report and submit it for verification.

1. Who are the third-party payers in May 2005?
2. What was the fill date for the One Touch Test Strips?
3. Are the One Touch Test Strips listed as OTC or Rx?

Quick Challenge

1 You are now familiar with the steps of generating a business report. Can you compile a *Profit Summary Report* for October 2005? Submit the printed report for verification.

Inventory Management

LAB OBJECTIVES

In this lab, you will:

- learn how to create a pharmacy business report that tracks pharmacy inventory. To gain a basic understanding of the concept of inventory, refer to Chapter 14 in Hopper, *Pharmacy Technician: Principles and Practice*.

Student Directions

Estimated completion time: 20 minutes

1. Read through the steps before performing the lab exercise on your computer.
2. After reading through the lab, perform the required steps to generate the inventory report and to adjust the electronic inventory records.
3. Complete the questions at the end of the lab.
4. Complete the exercise at the end of the lab.

Steps

1 Access the main screen of Visual SuperScript.

2 Click on **INVENTORY** on the menu toolbar located at the top of the screen.

3 Select **DRUG INVENTORY** from the expanded menu list.

4 Click on **PREVIEW** in the *Drug Inventory* pop-up box.

5 The *Drug Inventory Report* appears. This report consists of over 99 pages listing the drug, the drug NDC number, and the current stock or inventory the pharmacy has of the given medication.

6 Click on the **CLOSE PREVIEW** icon located at the top of the screen.

7 Click on **CLOSE** at the bottom of the *Drug Inventory* dialog box.

8 Click on **INVENTORY** on the menu toolbar located at the top of the screen.

9 Select **DRUG STOCK** from the expanded menu list.

10 A **Drug Stock** dialog box will appear. Click on the **Arrow** to the right of the **Type** data entry field. Select either **Add** or **Adjust**. These options will allow you to adjust electronic inventory records that do not match the physical inventory count. Selecting **Adjust** will subtract drug quantities from the electronic file. Selecting **Add** will allow you to add drug quantities to the electronic file.

Select *Adjust*.

11 Key in the **NDC** number of the medication that will be adjusted in the **Drug** data entry field.

Key in *00002-0363-33* as the NDC number for Darvocet N 100 tablets.

> **HINT:** To facilitate NDC data entry, right-click on the **Drug Data** entry field. Right-clicking on this field will enable a pick list *NDC Lookup* dialog box.

12 Key in a short comment relating to the adjustment or addition to the stock in the **Notes** data entry field.

Key in *"Correcting physical/electronic discrepancy."*

13 Key in the **Quantity** of medication that should be added (**Add**) or subtracted (**Adjust**) from the electronic file.

Key in *10*.

14 Enter the correct **Lot No.** (lot number) and **Exp. Date** (expiration date) from the drug label.

Enter *Lot # 256PO*. Enter *Expiration date: 10/2010*.

15 Check the **VERIFY STOCK** check box to indicate that a physical count took place.

16 Print the screen by using the **PRINTSCRN** option on your keyboard: Press the **PRINTSCRN** key, open a blank Word document, **RIGHT-CLICK** the blank Word document, and then select **PASTE**.

17 Click on **SAVE** located at the bottom of the *Drug Stock* dialog box.

18 Click on **CANCEL** to exit the *Drug Stock* task.

Questions for Review

1 According to the *Inventory Report*, how many Zyrtec D tablets are on hand?

2 What is the AWP cost for Acetaminophen with Codeine #4 tablet, NDC 51079-0106-20?

Exercise

Scenario

The pharmacy manager has put you in charge of the end-of-the-month task of pulling the outdated prescription medication off the shelf.

Task

Enter the physical inventory adjustments into the electronic database. Following is a list of outdated and soon-to-outdate medications that you pulled from the shelf. Submit the on-screen work for verification.

1. Zyprexa 7.5 mg tablet
NDC 00002-4116-60
Expiration date: 03/2007
Lot: N2369J
16 tablets remaining in the stock bottle that was pulled
from the shelf

2. Evista 60 mg tablet
NDC 00002-4165-02
Expiration date: 05/2007
Lot: 236MK8
23 tablets remaining in the stock bottle

Quick Challenge

1 You have learned how to access the *Drug Inventory Report* and
how to make adjustments to the electronic drug inventory records.
Can you access the *Drug Inventory Report* for the Darvocet N 100
that was adjusted in the preceding lab?

2 According to the Drug Inventory Report, what is the current stock
for the Darvocet N 100? What is the *total* current stock for
Darvocet N 100?

Refilling a Retail Prescription

LAB OBJECTIVES

In this lab, you will:

- learn how to refill a prescription
- create a new prescription out of an expired prescription
- learn the procedure in faxing the prescriber for additional refill requests
- learn how to generate a *Refill Reminder Report*

Student Directions

Estimated completion time: 45 minutes

1. Read through the steps before performing the lab exercise on your computer.
2. After reading through the lab, perform the required steps to refill a prescription.
3. Answer the questions at the end of the lab.
4. Complete the exercise at the end of the lab.

Steps

1 Access the main screen of Visual SuperScript. Click on *Options* on the top right of the menu screen and select *Workstation Setup*. Make sure the correct printer is selected.

2 Select **FILL RX'S** on the menu screen by clicking on the **FILL RX'S** icon.

3 The *Prescription Processing* form appears on your screen. Click on the **REFILL BY RX #** button located on the left side of the screen. It may be necessary to click on the **ARROW** next to the **REFILL RX'S** menu on the left of the form to access the expanded **REFILL RX'S** menu choices.

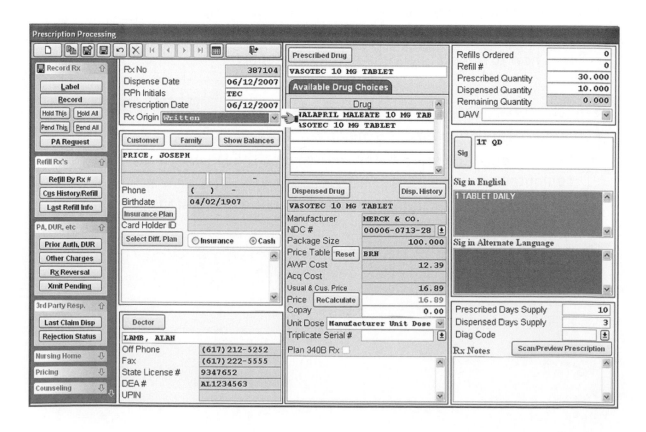

4 Key in the prescription number that is to be refilled in the **Rx No.** box.

> **Enter *201268* as the prescription refill number.**

5 The *Cannot Refill, Select Copy Options* dialog box appears. This dialog box will appear when a prescription has no refills remaining or if the prescription has expired.

6 Click on **REFILL AUTH REQUEST FORM** located on the right side of the dialog box. This will automatically generate and print a refill authorization form for the patient's medication. The refill authorization form may then be faxed to the patient's physician. (Be sure to have the **PRINT** option checked. The **PRINT** option is located directly below **REFILL AUTH REQUEST FORM**).

7 Click on **COPY TO NEW Rx** pad located at the bottom right of the *Cannot Refill, Select Copy Options* dialog box.

8 A series of dialog boxes will appear alerting you to *Price Increases* and/or *HIPAA*. Navigate through these dialog boxes by clicking on **OK** or **CLOSE**.

9 The *Prescription Processing* form appears and a new prescription is automatically created. This new prescription and subsequent refills will need to be authorized by the physician. (The refill authorization form in step 6 is used to authorize refills.)

10 Make note that the new prescription number and other prescription information is automatically added to the form.

11 Click on the **RPʜ Iɴɪᴛɪᴀʟs** data entry field. The data entry field is now highlighted in blue. Delete the text that is currently in the data entry field and key in your initials and your job title.

**Key in *TEC* for pharmacy technician
or *RP* for registered pharmacist.**

12 Click on the **Sᴀᴠᴇ** icon located at the top left of the screen.

13 Click on **Lᴀʙᴇʟ** at the top left of the form. The *Send Claim* dialog box pops up. The prescription label will print out when the claim is processed.

> **HINT:** Use the printed label to complete the refill process for this patient. Refer to your instructor for complete instructions.

Questions for Review

1 What is the sig on Joseph Price's prescription?

2 What company manufacturers the medication refilled in Joseph Price's prescription?

3 What is the price and the copay on the Vasotec prescription for Joseph Price?

4 What is the new prescription number that was created for Joseph Price's prescription?

Exercise

1 Follow the steps from the preceding lab to refill the following medication orders. Submit the labels for verification.

  a Brian Davidson's Pen-Vee K #201096

  b Fred Flintstone's Demadex #386530

  c Mary Harrison's Celebrex #386529

> **HINT:** When the prescription number is not given, use **Cus/History/Refill** located on the left side of the screen to access patient names and prescription information.

Quick Challenge

1 You have learned how to refill a retail prescription. Do you know how to make changes to the refill form?

  a Refill prescription #201171 for Carol Malone. The prescriber authorized an additional 2 refills for Ms. Malone's Coumadin. Submit the label for verification.

2 Can you access the *Refill Reminder List*?

  a Print a *Refill Reminder Letter* for Mattie Allen listing refills due from 04/01/2005 through 05/31/2005. Submit the *Refill Reminder Letter* for verification.

Steps to Refill Reminder List/Letter

1. Click on **Reports** from the Menu toolbar located at the top of the screen.
2. Select **Refill Reminders**, then **Refill Reminder List/Letter** from the expanded menu.
3. From the *Refill Reminder List/Letter* dialog box, select the appropriate **Paytype, Range of Dates, Range of Patients, Sort,** and **Select** formatting. Hint: If a letter is to be printed for only one patient, enter the patient's name in the **Patients Name From** and **To** fields.
4. Click on **Preview** or **Print**.

Entering a New Prescription

LAB OBJECTIVES

In this lab, you will:

- learn how to perform necessary computer functions to enter a new prescription into a pharmacy system
- learn about dispense as written (DAW) codes
- learn shortcuts to be used when entering sigs

Regardless of the practice setting for the pharmacy technician or the pharmacist, entering data into the computer is a major component of their workload. In the retail setting, for instance, a customer drops off the prescription hard copy. After the pharmacy technician has obtained all the necessary information from the customer, information is entered into the computer. This lab explains the steps involved in filling new prescriptions.

It is beneficial to work through the steps involved in interpreting and transcribing a prescription before completing the following lab.

Student Directions

Estimated completion time: 1 hour

1. Read through the steps before performing the lab exercise on your computer.
2. After reading through the lab, perform the required steps using the sample prescription.
3. Answer the questions at the end of the lab.
4. Complete the exercise at the end of the lab.

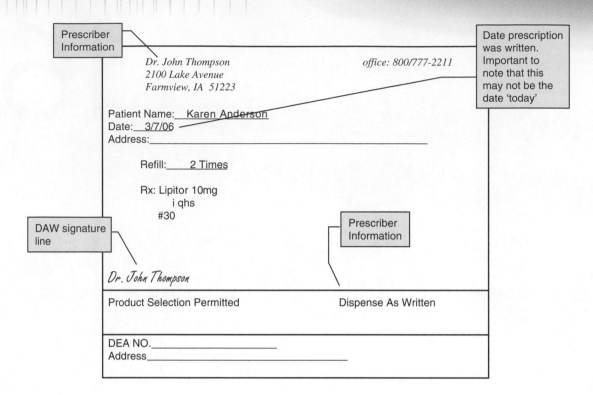

Prescriber Information

Dr. John Thompson
2100 Lake Avenue
Farmview, IA 51223

office: 800/777-2211

Date prescription was written. Important to note that this may not be the date 'today'

Patient Name:___Karen Anderson___
Date:___3/7/06___
Address:_____

Refill:_____2 Times___

Rx: Lipitor 10mg
      i qhs
      #30

DAW signature line

Prescriber Information

Dr. John Thompson

Product Selection Permitted   Dispense As Written

DEA NO._____
Address_____

Steps

Use the prescription above to complete the following steps.

1 Access the main menu of Visual SuperScript.

2 Click on **Fill Rx's** located on the left side of the menu screen.

3 The *Prescription Processing* form appears. Click on the **New Rx** icon [🗋] at the top left of the form.

4 Make note that prescription information such as the **Rx No.** (prescription number) and **Dispense Date** are automatically generated and added to the form.

5 You will then be prompted to the **Customer's Name** text box.

6 Press the **F3** key to bring up the customer database/pick list, which is entitled *Customer Lookup*.

7 Select the appropriate customer by double-clicking on customer name or by clicking on customer name and then clicking on **OK** at the bottom of the dialog box.

> **Select *Karen Anderson* as your customer as indicated in the sample Rx.**

8 The customer's personal information such as **ADDRESS**, **PHONE**, and **BIRTHDATE** will automatically be added to the *Prescription Processing* form.

9 Click on the **RPH INITIALS** data entry field. The data entry field is now highlighted in blue. Delete the text that is currently in the data entry field and key in your initials and your job title.

> **Enter *TEC* for pharmacy technician or *RP* for registered pharmacist.**

10 Press the **TAB** key. You will be then be prompted to the **DOCTOR** text box. For new prescriptions, the system will search the patient's prescription file to find the name of the prescriber of the most recently filled prescription. If found, the system will insert that name into this field. In case the new prescription is written by a different doctor, you can delete that name and enter a new one.

11 Press the **TAB** key. You will be prompted to the **PRESCRIBED DRUG** data entry field.

12 Key in the first three letters of the prescribed drug into the **PRESCRIBED DRUG** data entry field. Then press **ENTER**.

**Enter *Lip* for Karen Anderson's Lipitor.
Press ENTER.**

13 A drop-down list appears entitled *Drug Name Lookup*. Select the appropriate drug from the drop-down list by double-clicking on the drug name.

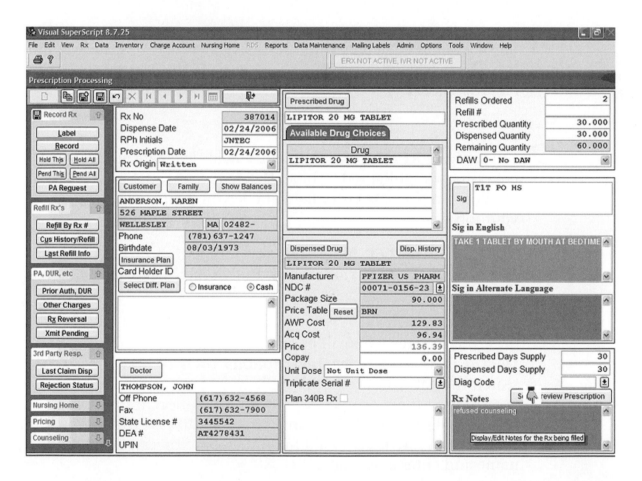

14 A series of warning dialog boxes will appear. Click **CLOSE** to move through warnings. Click **CONTINUE RX** to navigate to the next step. (The warning messages should be viewed and approved by the pharmacist before dispensing the medication.)

15 Double-click on the drug name a second time. The drug information such as **NDC#** and **Manufacturer** will be automatically added to the *Prescription Processing* form.

16 Next, you will be prompted to the **Refills Ordered** data entry field. Key in the appropriate number of refills.

When filling a prescription, it is necessary to know the correct **DAW** code to be assigned to a prescription for reimbursement. In order for this to be accomplished, distinguish between the brand name and the generic name of the medication. Although the prescriber may write the brand name of a drug on a patient's prescription, it may not necessarily mean that the brand-name drug must be dispensed. If the prescriber indicates DAW (dispense as written) or "brand name medically necessary" on the patient's prescription for a brand-name drug, the brand-name drug rather than the generic alternative MUST be dispensed. This situation, for example, would be a **DAW** code 1. The failure to use the proper DAW codes may result in improper third-party reimbursement to the pharmacy. There are seven DAW codes used in the practice of pharmacy:

DAW 0—Physician has approved the dispensing of a generic medication

DAW 1—Physician requests that the brand-name drug be dispensed

DAW 2—Physician has approved the dispensing of a generic drug, but the patient has requested that the brand-name drug be dispensed

DAW 3—Pharmacist dispense as written

DAW 4—No generics available in store

DAW 5—Brand dispensed, but priced as generic

DAW 6—RPh doctor call attempt

17 Press the **TAB** key. You will be prompted to enter the prescribed quantity. Key in the appropriate quantity in the **PRESCRIBED QUANTITY** data entry field.

18 Press the **TAB** key until you reach the **DAW** text box.

19 Choose the correct **DAW** code by clicking on the **ARROW** on the right side of the **DAW** data entry field. Click on the correct **DAW** code from the pick list.

20 Press the **TAB** key. Key in patient abbreviated directions in the **SIG** text box. If an error is made when typing in the sig, backspace to delete the error and retype the correct information.

Key in *T1T PO HS* as the shortcut abbreviation sig for Karen Anderson.

> **HINT:** Appendix A contains a complete listing of Visual SuperScript sig abbreviations.

21 Press the **TAB** key. You will be prompted to enter **PRESCRIBED DAYS SUPPLY**.

Days supply involves calculating the number of days that a particular prescription will last. All third-party payers require this information. The failure to provide days supply information properly may result in the pharmacy losing money. To calculate the days supply a prescription will last, use the following formula:

Days supply = total quantity dispensed/total quantity taken per day

The days supply is the number of days a medication will last for one filling. Days supply does not take into account refills. The majority of the third-party payers will reimburse a pharmacy for a 30-day supply of medication.

22 Key in the appropriate days supply in the **Prescribed Days Supply** data entry field.

> **Enter *30* for Karen Anderson's days supply.**

23 Key in comments in the **Rx Notes** section. Most states require patients to receive the opportunity for medication counseling. The **Rx Notes** section is a good spot to document "offered counseling, but patient refused counseling" or other such important information.

24 Press the **Tab** key. You are now prompted to save the prescription information. Click on the **Save** icon.

25 Click on **Label** on the left of the screen to complete adjudication.

Questions for Review

1 How is the data entry field identified when information is ready to be added?

2 What procedure do you follow to look up a new patient in the system?

3 How does the software prompt you to choose a generic equivalent?

4 What keyboard character separates the patient's last name from the first name?

5 Are you able to use shorthand when entering new prescription information? Explain by giving an example.

6 Click on the *Insurance Plan* tab on the fill screen for Karen Anderson. What is the plan name and company of Karen Anderson's insurance?

7 The section of the label that will be affixed to the medication vial or container includes

  a Patient name and address

  b Pharmacy name and address

  c Physician name and address

  d A and B only

  e all of the above

8 Using a highlight marker, highlight the following information on the prescription label that was generated in the preceding lab for Karen Anderson:

  a Pharmacy name, address, phone

  b Brand name of medication

  c Generic name of medication

  d NDC number

  e Prescription number

  f Patient education information

Exercise

Fill the following prescriptions. The second prescription for Betty Grace will require adding new patient information and new prescriber information to the database. Use the physician information provided on the written script to update the doctor database. Use the information on the insurance card to help update the customer profile. When completing this exercise, role-play with a classmate. Your classmate will role-play the customer, Betty Grace, giving you necessary information to update the customer profile.

Dr. William J. Smith   *office: 617-334-4455*
2315 Nassau St.
Allston, MA 02134

Patient Name:___Douglas Richards___
Date:___3/14/07___
Address:_____

    Refill:_____2 Times___

    Rx: Synthroid 0.025mg
        i q d
     #30

Dr. William Smith

Product Selection Permitted	Dispense As Written

DEA NO._____
Address_____

Dr. Susan Jonson   *office: 800/319-0862*
2319 Kidd Rd.
Glencity, IA 51263

Patient Name: Betty Grace
Date: 5/17/07
Address:_____

    Refill: 4 Times

    Rx: Tretinoin Cream 0.025%
        apply once qd a hs as directed
        #20 gm

Dr. Susan Johnson

Product Selection Permitted   Dispense As Written

DEA NO.   AJ1234592-014
Address_____
State License NO. 52368

Staywell Insurance

Grace, Betty   01
DOB: 1/10/1958
Insured Address: 109 Palm Lane
                    Hawaiian Village,
                    NE 68523
Insured Phone: 402/526-1319
Effective Date: 1/01/2007
ID#: **QT**9969

Pharmacy Information:
Submit electronic claims to Ameriscript
RxBIN: 610020
Group#4789521569

Quick Challenge

1 You have learned how to add a new prescription to the pharmacy software system. In Lab 4, you learned how to add a new customer to the database. Can you edit the patient information from the *Prescription Processing* screen?

   a Click on **Customer** on the *Prescription Processing* form to make patient information changes.

   b The patient in the preceding prescription, Betty Grace, is taking OTC Claritin 10 mg. Add this information to the *Customers* form via the *Prescription Processing* form.

   c Use the **PrintScrn** option on your keyboard to save the edited information for submission.

2 Appendix A has a listing of the abbreviated **Sig** codes for Visual SuperScript. Can you access the listing of **Sig** codes electronically?

   a Click on **Data** from the menu bar, then click on **Sig** from the expanded menu.

   b The *Sig* dialog box pops up. Click on the **List** icon for a complete electronic listing of sig abbreviations.

   c Write down the shortcut abbreviations for (i) as needed, (ii) left ear, and (iii) take one capsule three times a day.

   d Practice entering shortcut sig abbreviations in the **Sig** data entry field.

Filling and Refilling Tasks

LAB OBJECTIVES

In this lab, you will:

- learn how to perform daily tasks associated with filling a prescription
- learn how to refill a batch of prescriptions, how to transfer a prescription to another pharmacy, and how to put a prescription on file
- learn the accounting procedure for how to charge transactions (the Quick Challenge will guide you through this)

Student Directions

Estimated completion time: 1 hour

1. Read through the steps before performing the lab exercise on your computer.
2. After reading through the lab, perform the required steps to complete the tasks in each scenario.
3. Answer the questions at the end of the lab.

Batch Refill

Scenario

Mr. Ronald Jackson asks you to refill all of his medications for the month.

Task

Instead of entering each prescription number separately, *Batch Refill* allows for multiple refills. Refill Ronald Jackson's 2005 medications by following the *Steps to Batch Refill*.

Steps

Use the information box above to complete the following steps.

1 From the *Prescription Processing* form, click on the **ARROW** next to the **REFILL Rx's** menu on the left of the form to access the expanded **REFILL Rx's** menu.

2 Click on **CUS HISTORY/REFILL**.

3 Key the customer name into the **CUSTOMER** data entry field of the *Customer History: Refill Rx's* dialog box. Press the **ENTER** key. The *Customer Lookup* dialog box appears. Click on the correct customer from the list in the *Customer Lookup* dialog box. Click on **OK**.

Enter customer name JACKSON, RONALD.

4 Select the tab titled **PRESCRIPTIONS ON FILE**. Put a checkmark in the check box of the prescriptions that need to be refilled.

5 Click on **REFILL RX** located at the top of the dialog box.

6 If the prescription has *not* expired and there are refills remaining, the *Prescription Processing* form is updated with the refill information. If the prescription *has* expired, it may be necessary to click on **COPY TO NEW RX** from the *Cannot Refill, Select Copy Options* dialog box.

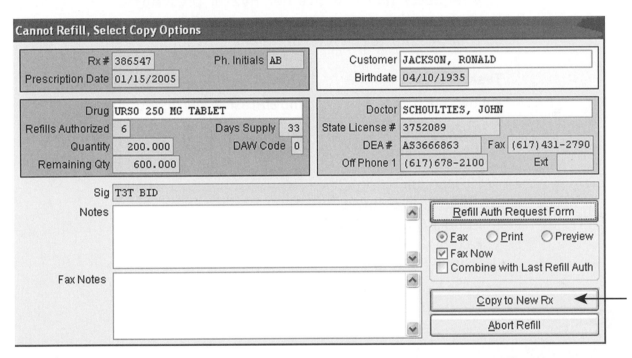

7 The *Prescription Processing* form now returns to the screen. All meds checked in the batch refill will process through. Click on **LABEL** located at the top left of the form. Clicking on **LABEL** will prompt the software to adjudication. Note: This educational version of Visual SuperScript will not allow adjudication. You will receive a message that electronic billing is not supported. Click *OK*. To print the labels, change the **PAY TYPE** to *Cash*.

Transferring a Prescription

Scenario

Mrs. Shirley Jones phones the pharmacy explaining that she is on vacation visiting her daughter in Phoenix, Arizona. Mrs. Jones is out of her Hyzaar. She requests that you give her Hyzaar prescription information to a nearby pharmacy in Phoenix, so that she may get a refill on the medication.

Task

Follow the *Steps to Transferring a Prescription* listed below in order to transfer Shirley Jones' prescription for Hyzaar to the following pharmacy:

 Sun Drug
 102 Indian School Rd.
 Phoenix, AZ 85025
 Phone: 602/321-9632
 Fax: 602/321-9633
 Fred Fixit RPh

Steps

Use the information box above to complete the following steps.

1 From the *Prescription Processing* form, click on the **ARROW** next to **MISC** (miscellaneous) located on the bottom left corner of the form.

2 Click on **XFER OUT** (transfer out). The *Customer History: Transfer Rx Out* dialog box pops up.

3 Key in the customer name in the **CUSTOMER** data entry field. Press the **ENTER** key. The *Customer Lookup* dialog box appears. Click on the appropriate customer from the lookup list and click on **OK**.

4 Put a check mark in the check box of the prescription that should be transferred to another pharmacy.

Customer History: Transfer Rx Out

Customer	JONES, SHIRLEY	Phone	(781) 333-4434	User Interface
Address	123 MAIN	Birthdate	10/17/1937	◉ Basic ○ Ad...

[**X**fer Out] [Cancel]

Prescriptions on File= 5, # Selected for Refills= 1

Refill History

R	Rx #	Pres Date	Prescribed Drug	Quantity	Rem Qty	Days Supply	Last Fill Date ☐	Last Disp. Qty	Doctor
☑	386545	01/15/2005	HYZAAR 50-12.5 TABLET	30.000	0.000	30	04/15/2005	30.000	NOBEL, ALFRED
☐	386652	02/09/2005	EFFEXOR XR 75 MG CAPSULE SA	30.000	0.000	30	04/10/2005	30.000	NOBEL, ALFRED
☐	386572	01/20/2005	SINGULAIR 10 MG TABLET	30.000	90.000	30	03/21/2005	30.000	NOBEL, ALFRED
☐	386718	03/06/2005	TAZORAC 0.1% CREAM	15.000	30.000	5	03/06/2005	15.000	NOBEL, ALFRED
☐	386559	01/18/2005	ALCOHOL SWABS	100.000	0.000	30	01/18/2005	100.000	NOBEL, ALFRED

Hot Keys | **M= Menu**

A= Show All	D= Show Selected Drug Only	R= Selected for Refills	H= Refill History	F= Fill Rx
S= Sort On Prescribed / Dispensed Date	E= Edit Prescription	I= Inactivate Rx	T= Transfer Rx Out	

[Show All] [Selected Drug] [Selected For Refills] [Drug]

5 Click on **Xfer Out** located at the top of the dialog box.

6 At this time, you will verbally relay the prescription information to the pharmacist or pharmacy technician at the pharmacy that the prescription is being transferred to. Although the prescription transfer is noted on the customer records, the actual transfer of the prescription information does not occur electronically. It is necessary to speak with the other pharmacy in order to relay prescription information. Many states require a pharmacist, only, to transfer prescriptions and to accept transferred prescriptions.

7 Complete the *Transfer Rx Out* dialog box information. Click on **Transfer Rx** located at the bottom of the dialog box.

8 Print the screen by using the **PrintScrn** option on your keyboard. Press the **PrintScrn** key, open a blank Word document, right-click the blank Word document, and then select **Paste**.

Steps to Transfer a Prescription

Transfer of prescription information between pharmacies in most states is communicated directly between two licensed pharmacists. The *transferring* pharmacist enters/records the following:

- Name, address, and registration number of the pharmacy to which the prescription was transferred.
- Date of transfer and the name of the pharmacist transferring the information, as well as the pharmacist receiving the information.
- The pharmacist *receiving* the transferred prescription information enters/records the following:
- Date of issuance of original prescription, original number of refills authorized, date of original dispensing, number of valid refills remaining, and dates and locations of previous refills.
- Pharmacy name, address, registration number, and prescription number from which the prescription information was transferred.
- Name of the pharmacist who transferred the prescription and pharmacy name, address, registration number, and prescription number from which the prescription was originally filled.
- Certain restrictions apply to the transferring of prescription information for Schedule III-V controlled substances.

Putting a Prescription on File

Scenario

Mrs. Carla Watson is at the pharmacy this afternoon with two prescriptions from the dentist. One prescription is for an antibiotic and the other is for pain medication. Mrs. Watson would like to have the antibiotic filled, but she is not sure that she needs the pain medication. "I really have no pain," she explains, "I hate to take the pain pills if I don't need them. Can you keep the prescription for pain pills in case I start having pain later this evening or tomorrow morning?"

Task

Put Mrs. Carla Watson's prescription for pain medication on file. Putting the prescription on file will electronically store the prescription for Mrs. Watson without charging her insurance company or filling the order.

Kally Luck DDS
1324 Lady Luck Street
Las Vegas, NV 90215

office: 717-333-8996
fax: 717-333-8990

Patient Name: Carla Watson   Date: 7/07/2007

Address:_____

                                         Refill: 0 Times

Rx: Tylenol c codeine #3
     i-ii po prn pain
     #10

Kally Luck

Product Selection Permitted	Dispense As Written

DEA NO. BL24681352

Address_____

State License: 45231

Steps

Use the information on the previous page to complete the following steps.

1 From the *Prescription Processing* form, complete the patient/ prescription information just as you would if you were filling a new prescription.

2 After the *Prescription Processing* form is completed, click on **HOLD THIS** located at the top left corner of the form.

3 A label will be generated even though this medication will not be filled. A section of the label will be filed with the prescription hard copy for record-keeping purposes.

4 Click on **CUS HISTORY/REFILL** located on the left side of the screen. Check to be sure that the prescription has been put on file.

5 A prescription that has been put on file or on hold can be filled at a later date by accessing the prescription from the *Customer History/Refill Rx's* form.

Questions for Review

1 Why is a prescription put *on file*?

2 Prescriptions may only be transferred out of the pharmacy. Accepting *transferred in* prescriptions is against the law.

   a True

   b False

Quick Challenge

1 You have learned how to perform many fill and refill functions. Do you know how to charge a prescription?

2 Take the preceding prescription for Carla Watson off file and fill it. Charge the Tylenol prescription to Mrs. Watson by following the *Charging Prescription Steps*. Submit the *Charge Account Transaction Report* for verification.

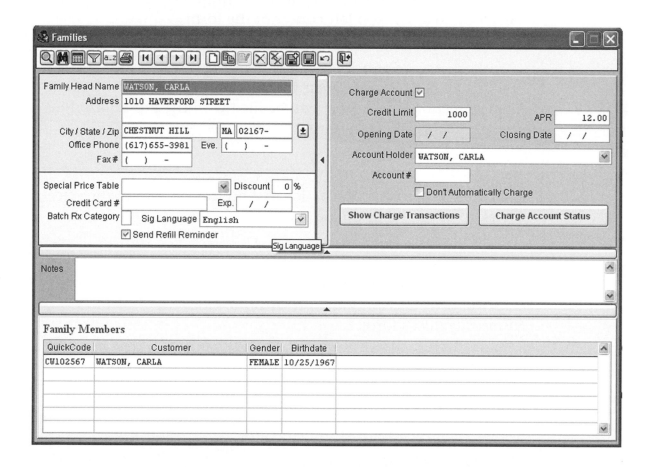

Charging Prescription Steps

1 From the *Customer* form, access the **FAMILY HEAD** information form.

2 Edit the *Families* form to confirm that the customer has a **Charge Account**. It may be necessary to add the customer to the **Account Holder** table.

3 **Save** and **Close** both the *Families* form and the *Customers* form.

4 Click on **Charge Account** from the menu toolbar.

5 Click on **Charge Transactions** from the menu list.

6 Click on the **New** icon. Key in the required information in the *Charge Transactions* dialog box.

7 Be sure to choose **Charge** from the list of options in the **Type** data entry field.

8 Key in the prescription number in the **Ref#** field.

9 Click on the **Save** icon at the top of the dialog box.

10 Click on **Charge Account** from the menu toolbar.

11 Click on **Charge Transaction List** from the menu list.

12 Key in the required information in the *Charge Transactions List* dialog box.

13 Select **SINGLE** from the **FAMILY SELECTION** and key in the family name.

14 Click on **PREVIEW** to view the report before printing/submitting.

NURSING HOME

Adding a New Patient and New Orders

LAB OBJECTIVES

In this lab, you will:

- learn how to enter a new nursing home patient and nursing home orders into the software system. You will find that entering nursing home information is very similar to entering ambulatory customer information with a few additional steps.

Student Directions

Estimated completion time: 1 hour

1. Read through the steps before performing the lab exercise on your computer.
2. After reading through the lab, perform the required steps to process a nursing home order by using the sample physician order.
3. Complete the review questions.

PHYSICIAN ORDERS

Patient Name: Fred C. Wilson
Allergies: PCN, MSO4
DOB: 08/26/1930
                   Milk
SSN: 480-25-7117
Sex: Male
Primary Insurance: Medicare Plan D-Wellcare
    ID: Medicare D 109A
    Group: Medicare D
    Member: 00

4/4/2007
0800
Admit to Coolidge Corner Nursing Home per Dr. John Adams.
Dx: dementia, beginning episodes of Alzheimer's disease.
Labs: weekly CBC
Diet: DAT
Patient may smoke 1 cigar after evening meal if desires.   *John Adams*

Coolidge Corner Nursing Home
4560 Beacon St.
Brookline, MA 02446   #617-555-1212

Patient Care Notes

Mr. Wilson Admitted on 4/4/2007 to room 41A.
Dr. Adams has asked nursing to obtain a list of current
medications from patient.

Steps

1 Access the main screen of Visual SuperScript.

2 Click on the **CUSTOMERS** icon located on the left side of the screen.

3 A dialog box entitled *Customers* will pop up.

4 Click on the **FIND** icon, which is located at the top left of the *Customers* dialog box toolbar.

5 A dialog box entitled *Customer Lookup* pops up. Enter the first letter of the customer's last name into the **NAME** data entry field. Scroll through the *Customer Lookup* pop-up table to be certain that the customer is not in the database.

> **HINT:** Use the vertical scroll bar located on the right side of the pop-up box to view customer information.

6 The customer name is not located in the *Customer Lookup* table. Click on **ADD** located at the bottom of the *Customer Lookup* dialog box.

7 A dialog box entitled *Customers* pops up. The *Customers* dialog box contains four tabbed forms. Click on the tab entitled *Customer*.

8 The form is now ready to enter new patient information.

9 The **NAME** is a required field and allows up to 30 characters. The recommended format is last name followed by a comma, a single space, first name, a single space, and middle initial or name (if known). Example: Johnson, Linda P.

> **Enter *Fred C. Wilson* from the physician order sheet.**

> **HINT:** To facilitate searching your database, it is very important that you follow the recommended format for entering names.

10 The format for entering the **BIRTHDATE** is mm/dd/yyyy. Example: 05/10/1998 (do not enter as 5/10/1998).

Enter Fred C. Wilson's date of birth (DOB) from the physician order sheet.

11 **Q CODES** (Quick Codes) allow you to expedite the search for customers when filling prescriptions. Enter the patient's initials in this field.

12 **PAY TYPE** is a very important field. It determines how prescriptions filled for this patient are priced and who is expected to pay for them. Two **PAY TYPES** are permissible: Private and Insurance. Click on the ARROW located to the right of the **PAY TYPE** data entry field. Make the appropriate selection.

13 Click on the **ARROW** located to the right of the **GENDER** data entry field. Make the appropriate selection.

14 Click on the **ARROW** located to the right of the **SMOKING** data entry field. Make the appropriate selection from the list.

15 The next data entry field is the **PATIENT IDENTIFICATION** field. The state government or the pharmacy may require additional patient identification information. Click on the **ARROW**. A drop-down list appears with patient ID choices. Click on the appropriate choice.

16 Tab to the **FIRST VISIT DATE** and **LAST VISIT DATE** fields. These fields contain the date of the most recent prescription filled for the customer. It is automatically updated while filling prescriptions, so you do not have to enter any value in it manually.

17 The **MTD RX Count** field contains the month-to-date count of the number of prescriptions filled for this customer. It is automatically updated while filling prescriptions, so you do not have to enter any value in it manually.

18 **Child-Proof Lid:** By default, this box will be checked for every customer that is added to the database, because the law requires the use of such a lid unless specified otherwise. If a customer desires easy-open lids, make sure to uncheck this box. In that case, the words "EZ CAP" will appear on the hard-copy segment of the prescription label as a reminder. The **Child-Proof Lid** section of the form will not be relevant to the nursing home patient unless the patient is discharged from the nursing home for a period of time.

19 **Duplicate Label:** Check this box if the customer requests two labels at the time the prescription for this patient is filled. This field will not be relevant for the nursing home customer/patient.

20 Tab to the **HIPAA Conf Statement** data entry field. Click in the check-off box to indicate that the patient has received HIPAA information. It is necessary for all customers to receive HIPAA statements. A family member of the nursing home resident may acknowledge receipt of the HIPAA statement.

21 Tab to the **Family** data entry field. The last name of the new customer is automatically entered into the **Family** data entry field. Press **Enter**. A box entitled *Family Head Lookup* pops up. Click on **Add** to add the family head.

22 The *Families* dialog box appears on the screen. **Family Head Name** is a required field and allows up to 30 characters. The recommended format is last name followed by a comma, a single space, first name, a single space, and middle initial or name (if known). Example: Wilson, Fred C.

HINT: To facilitate searching your database, it is very important that you follow the correct naming procedures.

23 Enter **Address** and **Phone** information for the nursing home patient. This will be the address and phone information of the nursing home itself, unless the customer specifically asks to have an alternate address listed. You may wish to include the name of the nursing home on the first line of the **Address** data entry field.

24 Tab to the **Notes** section. It may be necessary to click on the **Arrow** in order to access the **Notes** section of the form. This field will store reminders that apply to the nursing home patient. For instance, you may indicate the name of the family member(s) to contact with billing questions. Click in the **Notes** data entry field. The white field turns blue when ready to accept information.

Enter a short note in this field.

25 Tab to the account section of the form. It may be necessary to click on the **Arrow** located on the right side in order to access the account section.

26 Nursing home patients make use of charge accounts. Each month the nursing home resident and/or their designee receive a statement from the pharmacy that lists medication charges. Check the **Charge Account** check box as nursing home patients make use of charge accounts.

27 Specify a credit limit for the patient by keying a dollar amount into the **Credit Limit** data entry field. When filling prescriptions, Visual Superscript will warn you if the total unpaid balance exceeds the specified credit limit. Note: The default credit limit is $1000.00 with a 12% interest rate.

28 The **APR** data entry field is the annual percentage rate for finance charges to be applied to overdue balances. Key in a percentage amount, if the pharmacy desires to charge interest on account balances.

29 Tab to the **ACCOUNT HOLDER** data entry field. The account holder for the nursing home patient will be the party responsible for paying the monthly bill. To add the account holder name, press the **F2** key. Click on **ADD**. Update the *Account Holders* dialog box by keying in the appropriate information. Click on the **SAVE** icon. Click on the **CLOSE** icon. The account holder information has now been added to the database.

30 Tab through the remaining data entry fields on the *Families* form. Key in necessary information.

31 Click on the **SAVE** icon located on the toolbar at the top right of the *Families* dialog box. Then click on the **CLOSE** icon located on the toolbar at the top right of the *Families* dialog box. The family head of household information has now been added to the database. The *Customers* dialog box is again active and ready for the form to be completed.

32 Click on the **ARROW** located to the right of the **LOCATION CODE** data entry field. Choose **NURSING HOME** from the drop-down list.

33 Click on the **COMBO-BOX ARROW** next to the **NURSING HOME** data entry field. A list of nursing homes appears. Make the appropriate selection from the list. Click on **OK**.

34 Click on the **COMBO-BOX ARROW** next to the **PRIMARY MD** data entry field. A list of physicians appears. Make the appropriate selection from the list. Click on **OK**.

35 Tab to the **Notes** field. In this field you can enter whatever information you want to store about the nursing home patient. For instance, you may indicate any patient allergies that are not medication-type allergies. The information will appear on the *Prescription Processing Screen* as a reminder when filling a prescription for this patient.

Enter a short note in this field.

36 The bottom half of the *Customers* form contains many tabs. Click on the **Allergies** tab.

37 Click on the **Add a New Record** icon located on the bottom right of the *Customers* form. An *Allergy Lookup* table pops up. Make the appropriate selection(s).

38 Click on the **Other Drugs** tab. This grid contains information about other drugs that the patient is currently taking. These may be prescription drugs that were purchased from a different pharmacy, or they may be over-the-counter (OTC) drugs.

39 Click on the **Add a New Record** icon located at the bottom right of the *Customers* form. Press the **Enter** key to access a list of drugs. A *Drug Name Lookup* table pops up.

Enter *Aspirin child 81 mg TAB CHEW* as other drug.

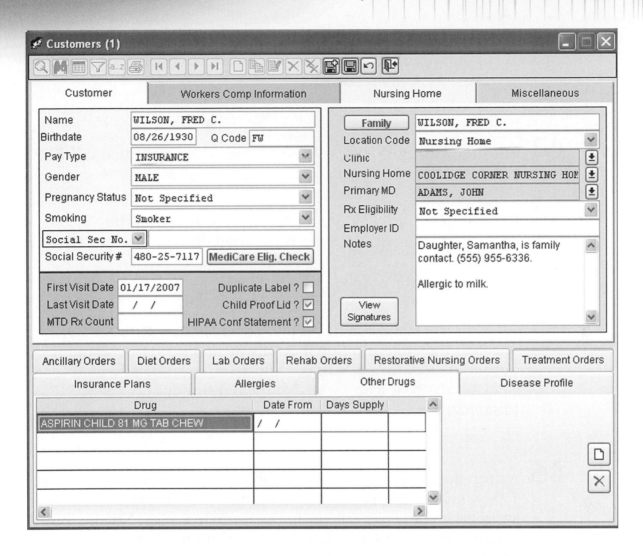

40 Look up the drug by typing the name of the drug in the **Name** dialog box. Click on the desired drug to select. Click on **OK**. Most often, nursing home patients will have all of their medications filled by the same pharmacy. Therefore the pharmacy will have a record of these medications, and it is not necessary to complete the **Other Drugs** information.

41 Click on the **Disease Profile** tab. This grid contains a list of diseases the customer has been diagnosed for. The information contained in this grid is used to check for drug-disease contraindications each time a prescription is filled for the patient.

42 Click on the **ADD A NEW RECORD** icon located at the bottom right of the *Customers* form. A red bar appears across the *Disease Profile* table.

43 Press the **F2** key. A *Disease Lookup* table pops up entitled *CFDBDX*.

44 Look up the disease by typing the first few letters of the name of the disease. Click on the desired disease to select. Click on **OK**.

45 Click on the **INSURANCE PLANS** tab. The insurance **PAYTYPE** is selected, therefore additional details such as Insurance Plan, Cardholder ID, Group Number, and so on must be provided. Click on the **NEW** icon located at the bottom right of the *Customers* form.

46 A drop-down list appears on the table under the heading *Coverage Type*. Click on the **ARROW** to the right of the list and choose the appropriate coverage type from the drop-down list. Nursing home patients, just as other patients, may have more than one insurance plan coverage. Select **PRIMARY** for the insurance plan that provides the main drug benefit coverage.

47 Press the **TAB** key and a new pick list appears entitled *Insurance*. Select the appropriate insurance plan. Click on **OK**.

48 Enter the **CARDHOLDER ID, GROUP NUMBER,** and **MEMBER NUMBER.**

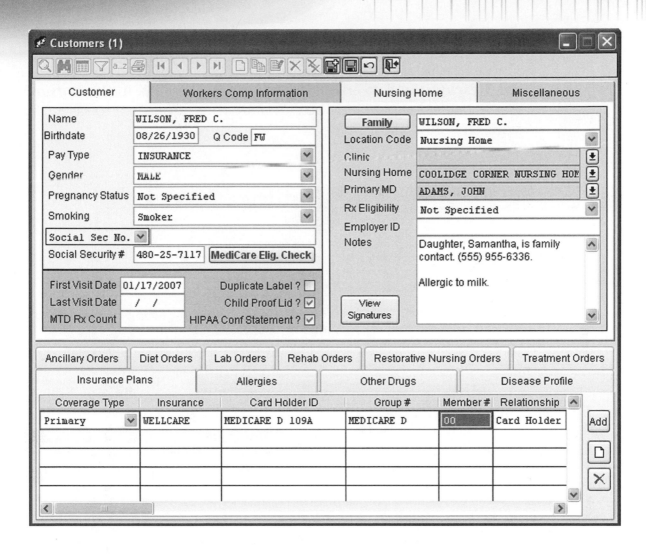

49 The Physicians' Orders for the nursing home patient may be grouped into six different categories: Ancillary Orders, Diet Orders, Lab Orders, Rehab Orders, Restorative Nursing Orders, and Treatment Orders. Click on the **LAB ORDERS** tab.

50 Click on the **ADD A NEW RECORD** icon located at the bottom right of the *Customers* form. The **ORDER DATE** is automatically added to the form. Tab to the **ORDER** data entry field. Press the **F2** key to bring up the *Order* dialog box.

51 Click on **Add** in the *Order* dialog box to add necessary lab orders. Choose *Lab Orders* for the **Order Type**. Then key in the order in the **Description** data entry field. Click on the red **X** in the *Nursing Home Doctor Orders* dialog box. You are then prompted to save your changes. Click on **Yes**.

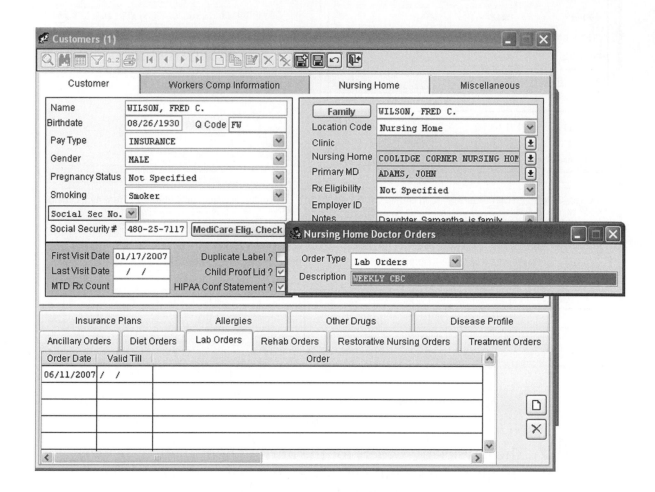

HINT: After you click on *Save*, you may need to click the *Edit* icon on the *Customers* toolbar to continue with adding diet orders.

52 Click on the **Diet Orders** tab.

53 Click on the **Add a New Record** icon located at the bottom right of the *Customers* form. The **Order Date** is automatically added to the form. Tab to the **Order** data entry field. Press the **F2** key to bring up the *Order* dialog box.

54 Click on **Add** in the *Order* dialog box to add necessary diet orders. Choose *Diet Orders* for the **Order type**. Then key in the order in the **Description** data entry field. Click on the red **X** in the *Nursing Home Doctor Orders* dialog box. You are then prompted to save your changes. Click on **Yes**.

55 Follow the same procedure used for **Diet Orders and Lab Orders for Ancillary orders, Restorative Orders, Treatment Orders**, and **Rehab Orders** (rehabilitation orders). Ancillary Orders may consist of physician orders that do not fit into the other given categories of order choices.

56 Click on the **Nursing Home** tab at the top of the form. Using the physician order sheet and information collected from the nursing home and the patient's family, update as much information in the *Nursing Home* section of the form as possible.

57 Click on the **Save** icon located at the top right of the toolbar.

58 Print the screen by using the **PrintScrn** option on your keyboard: Press the **PrintScrn** key, open a blank Word document, right-click the blank Word document, and then select **Paste**. Submit *Customer, Nursing Home*, and *Family Head* tabbed areas of the form, as well as the tabs at the bottom of the form where information was added (allergies, insurance, lab orders, etc.).

59 The new nursing home patient has now been added to the database.

60 Click the **Close** icon located at the top right of the toolbar.

Questions for Review

1 The Physicians' Orders may be grouped into six different categories: Ancillary Orders, Diet Orders, Lab Orders, Rehab Orders, Restorative Nursing Orders, and Treatment Orders.

   a True

   b False

2 When adding a new order, each order record contains three fields: the Order Type, the Order Date, and the Detailed Description of the order.

   a True

   b False

3 An example of an Ancillary Order may be:

   a Walk patient TID

   b Limit to 1 cup of coffee with each meal

   c Both a and b

   d Patient may attend mass every Sunday

Quick Challenge

1 You have learned how to add a new nursing home patient to the database. Can you add a nursing home to the database?

Steps to Add a Nursing Home to the Database

a Access the main screen of Visual Superscript.

b Click on the **NURSING HOME** option from the menu toolbar. Then click on **NURSING HOME** from the menu.

c Click on the **NEW** icon in the *Nursing Homes* dialog box. The dialog box is now ready to accept the **NAME, ADDRESS,** and **PHONE** information of the nursing home. Update the nursing home information by keying in the correct data.

d Click on the **SAVE** icon in the *Nursing Home* dialog box. Click on the **CLOSE** icon.

e You may verify that the nursing home information has been added to the database by clicking on the **LIST** icon in the *Nursing Home* dialog box. A list of current nursing homes will be displayed.

2 Add **Afton Heights Nursing Home. Create your own address and phone information. Submit the form for verification.**

Entering New Medication Orders

LAB OBJECTIVES

In this lab, you will:

- learn how to perform necessary computer functions to enter new medication orders for a nursing home patient
- learn how to print a nursing home Medication Record. The Quick Challenge teaches you how to compile an MAR (Medication Administration Record) for nursing home patients.

Student Directions

Estimated completion time: 1 hour

1. Read through the steps before performing the lab exercise on your computer.
2. After reading through the lab, perform the required steps using the sample Physician's Order sheet.
3. Complete the exercise at the end of the lab.

```
                         PHYSICIAN ORDERS


Patient Name:      Fred C. Wilson
Allergies:         PCN, MSO4
DOB:               08/26/1930
                   Milk
SSN:               480-25-7117
Sex:               Male
Primary Insurance: Medicare Plan D-Wellcare
          ID:      Medicare D 109A
          Group:   Medicare D
          Member:  00
4/5/2007
1030
Resume at home medications:
Aricept 5mg i tab po qhs
Lasix 40mg i po qam
Gemfibrozil 600mg i tab po 30' ac morning and evening meals
Colace 50mg ii caps po prn constipation
Valerian Herbal 500mg i po qhs                John Adams
```

Steps

1 Access the main menu of Visual SuperScript.

2 Click on **FILL RX'S** icon located on the left side of the menu screen.

3 The *Prescription Processing* form appears. Click on the **NEW RX** icon at the top left of the form.

4 Make note that prescription information such as the **RX No** (prescription number) and **DISPENSE DATE** are automatically generated and added to the form.

5 You will then be prompted to the **CUSTOMER'S NAME** text box.

6 Key in the first few letters of the patient's last name. Press **ENTER** to bring up the customer database/pick list, which is entitled *Customer Lookup*.

7 Select the appropriate customer by double-clicking on customer name or by clicking on customer name and then clicking on **OK** at the bottom of the dialog box.

8 The customer's personal information such as **ADDRESS**, **PHONE**, and **BIRTHDATE** will automatically be added to the *Prescription Processing* form.

9 You are prompted to the **DOCTOR** text box. For new prescriptions, the system will search the patient's prescription file to find the name of the prescriber of the most recently filled prescription. If the prescriber found, the system will insert that name into this field. In case the new prescription is written by a different doctor, you can delete that name and enter a new one.

10 You will be prompted to the **PRESCRIBED DRUG** data entry field.

11 Key in the first three letters of the prescribed drug into the **PRESCRIBED DRUG** data entry field. Then press **ENTER**.

12 A drop-down list appears entitled *Drug Name Lookup*. Select the appropriate drug from the drop-down list by double-clicking on the drug name.

13 A series of warning dialog boxes will appear. Click on **CONTINUE Rx** to navigate to the next step. (The warning messages should be viewed and approved by the pharmacist before dispensing the medication).

14 Double-click on the drug name that was entered in step 13. The drug name will be highlighted in red. The drug information such as **NDC#** and **MANUFACTURER** will be automatically added to the *Prescription Processing* form.

15 Click on the **RPh INITIALS** data entry field. The data entry field is now highlighted. **DELETE** the text that is currently in the data entry field and key in your initials and your job title.

16 Next, click on the **REFILLS ORDERED** data entry field. Nursing home patients are admitted to the care facility with a running order for their medications. This means that refills are permitted for 12 months on each prescription. However, most nursing home patients are covered by Medicaid and/or Medicare. Medicaid usually allows no more than 5 refills at a time. Additionally, Medicaid does not allow prescriptions to be refilled more than 6 months after the original prescription date. Key in the appropriate number of refills.

Enter 5 refills.

17 Press the **TAB** key. You will be prompted to enter the prescribed quantity. Nursing home patients are billed on a monthly cycle. The pharmacy calendar denotes 32 days in each month. Key in the appropriate quantity in the **PRESCRIBED QUANTITY** data entry field.

18 The *Prescription Processing* form automatically assumes and updates the **DISPENSED QUANTITY** to be the same as the prescribed quantity. If this is not the case, key in the quantity actually dispensed.

19 The **REMAINING QUANTITY** field is automatically updated. The value for this field is based on prescribed quantity, number of refills ordered, and the dispensed quantity.

20 Press the **Tab** key until you reach the **DAW** text box. Review **DAW** information in Lab 16, if necessary.

21 Choose the correct **DAW** code by clicking on the **Arrow** on the right side of the **DAW** data entry field. It is most appropriate to enter **DAW** code **0—No DAW** for nursing home orders. Click on the correct **DAW** code from the drop-down list.

22 Press the **Tab** key. Key in patient abbreviated directions in the **Sig** text box, which is highlighted in blue. If an error is made when typing in the sig, backspace to delete the error and retype the correct information.

Enter *T1T PO HS* as the shortcut abbreviation sig for Mr. Wilson's Aricept.

HINT: Appendix A contains a complete listing of Visual Superscript sig abbreviations.

23 Press the **Tab** key. You will be prompted to enter **Prescribed Days Supply**. A computed value based on the **Prescribed Quantity** entered in step 17 is automatically added to this field. You may override this value if necessary. Key in the appropriate days supply in the **Prescribed Days Supply** data entry field.

Days supply involves calculating the number of days that a particular prescription will last. All third-party payers require this information. The failure to provide days supply information properly may result in the pharmacy losing money. To calculate the days supply a prescription will last, use the following formula:

days supply = total quantity dispensed/total quantity taken per day

The days supply is the number of days a medication will last for one filling. Days supply does not take into account refills. The majority of third-party payers will reimburse a pharmacy for a 30-day supply of medication.

24 A few insurance plans require diagnosis information. Click on the **Combo-box Arrow** by the **Diag Code** (diagnosis code) data entry field. Select the appropriate diagnosis by clicking anywhere in the shaded diagnosis area of the table. Then key in the first letter of the diagnosis. The table will bring up relevant diagnoses. Double-click on the disease/diagnosis name.

25 Key in comments in the **Rx Notes** section.

26 Press the **Tab** key. You are now prompted to save the prescription information. Click on **Save Rx in System Memory and Start a New One for Same Customer.**

27 The *Batch Refill Information* dialog box appears. It is important to key in or select the required information in this box.

28 Click on the **Combo-box Arrow** to access a table of choices for **Batch Status**. Double-click on **B—Active Status**, as the nursing home patient is presently receiving medications.

29 Key in the **Daily Dosage**. This is the actual dosage amount that the nursing home patient will receive for the day.

Enter *5.00* for Mr. Wilson's Aricept to represent 5 mg.

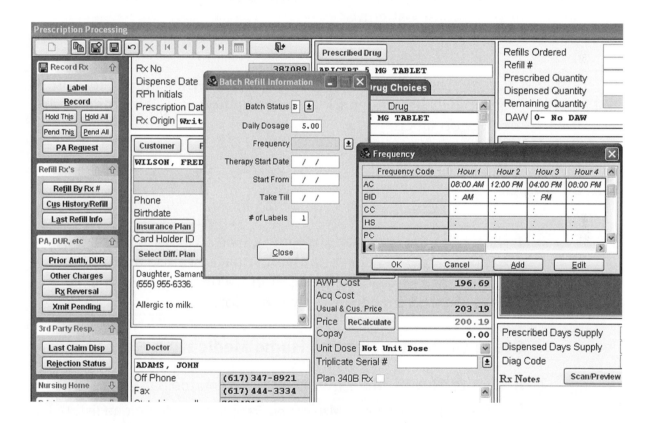

30 Click on the **Combo-box Arrow** to access a table of choices for **Frequency**. Double-click on the appropriate **Frequency** code. This information is very important to ensure that the nursing staff administers medication to the nursing home patient at the prescribed time of day.

31 Key in the medication **Therapy Start Dates**.

32 Click on **Close**.

33 You are now prompted to enter a new prescription for Fred C. Wilson.

34 Follow steps 10 through 32 to enter all medication orders for the nursing home patient.

35 Click on **Close** at the top left of the screen when all medication orders have been added for the nursing home patient to print all medication labels.

Exercise

1. Enter the five medications for Mr. Fred C. Wilson, as seen on the Physician Order sheet on the first page of this lab.
2. Print a Nursing Home Medication Record for Mr. Fred C. Wilson. Submit the record for verification.

Steps to Print a Nursing Home Medication Record

a Click on **Nursing Home** from the Main Menu toolbar.

b Click on **Nursing Home Medication Record** from the menu list.

c Key in the required information in the *Medication Record* dialog box.

d Preview the record before printing.

HINT: Press the **F2** key to access a list of nursing homes.

HINT: Use a 1-year time span for the **DATE FROM** and **To** fields.

Quick Challenge

1 You have learned how to add a new nursing home medication order to the pharmacy software system. You have also practiced generating a nursing home report, the Nursing Home Medication Report. Can you print an MAR? The MAR is a **M**edication **A**dministration **R**ecord. Among other items, the MAR lists medication name and dosing schedule. The nursing personnel at the care facility follow the MAR in order to administer patient medications at the correct times.

2 Print an MAR for Mr. Fred C. Wilson. Submit the record for verification.

   a Click on **NURSING HOME** from the main menu toolbar.

   b Click on **BATCH MAR PRINTING ON PLAIN PAPER** from the menu list.

   c Key in the required information in the *Batch MAR Printing on Plain Paper* dialog box. Hint: Select **ONE** in the **PRINT** section. Use today's date in the **MAR CHARTING To** field.

   d Preview the record before printing.

Cycle Refill

LAB OBJECTIVES

In this lab, you will:

- learn how to activate the refill cycle for nursing home medication orders
- be instructed to fill the nursing home cassettes by using the batch refill labels that you have generated

Student Directions

Estimated completion time: 25 minutes

1. Read through the steps before performing the lab exercise on your computer.
2. After reading through the lab, perform the required steps.
3. Complete the exercise at the end of the lab.
4. Answer the questions at the end of the lab.

The long-term care pharmacy will fill medication orders for a number of patients who reside at the nursing home. The nursing home, for example, may have 250 patients (also referred to as residents). Nursing home medication orders are refilled in cycles. Most long-term care pharmacies will refill nursing homes medication orders on a bimonthly cycle. This means that every 2 weeks the long-term care pharmacy will process a 2-week supply of medications for the nursing home residents/patients. The 2-week supply will then be delivered to the nursing home for patient administration.

Refilling nursing home medication orders in cycles is also referred to as batch refill. The first step in batch refill is to enter any new prescriptions into the system. Along with entering new orders, some prescriptions may have expired since the last refill, so it is important to generate new prescriptions for all expired ones. Once new prescriptions have been entered in the system it is necessary to make any changes requested by the nursing home. For instance, the nursing home may request that the administration time of a particular patient medication be changed from morning to evening. These changes must be noted on the electronic *Prescription* form.

Steps

Batch Refill

1 Click on **NURSING HOME** from the Main Menu toolbar.

2 Click on **BATCH REFILL RX'S** from the menu list.

3 The *Prescription Processing* form appears along with the *Batch Rx Refill* dialog box.

4 To activate the *Batch Rx Refill* dialog box, click in the **NURSING HOME** data entry field of the *Batch Rx Refill* dialog box. Press the **F2** key to bring up the *Nursing Home Lookup* table. Double-click on the nursing home name to select the appropriate nursing home.

Select *Coolidge Corner Nursing Home.*

5 Key in the appropriate **FILL DATE**. This is the date that the batch refills are processed by the pharmacy.

Enter *02/01/2006* as the fill date.

6 The **DAYS SUPPLY** will automatically be updated to correspond with the number of days in the month for the fill date in step 5.

7 Key in your initials and title (if different than RPh) in the **RPH INITIALS** data entry field.

8 Click on **OK**.

9 A *Confirmation* box pops up. Click on **OK** to *Proceed with Batch Refill.*

10 A dialog box will pop up to inform you of the number of prescriptions that were refilled. Click on **OK**.

11 Click on the **CLOSE** icon to close out the *Prescription Processing* form.

Print Batch Labels

1 Click on **OPTIONS** from the Main Menu toolbar.

2 Click on **RX LABEL OPTIONS** from the menu list.

3 Click on the **LABEL TYPE** data entry field **ARROW**.

4 Select **OPUS** from the list of label options.

5 Click on **OK**. The correct label format has now been selected for nursing home cassette filling.

6 Click on **NURSING HOME** from the Main Menu toolbar.

7 Click on **BATCH RX LABELS PRINTING** from the menu list.

8 The *Batch Rx Labels Printing* dialog box appears. Press the **F2** key to bring up the *Nursing Home Lookup* table. Double-click on the nursing home name to select the appropriate nursing home.

Select *Mass Elderly Care Home.*

9 Key in the appropriate **FILL DATE**. This is the date that the batch refills are processed by the pharmacy.

Enter *02/01/2006* for the fill date.

10 The labels may be sorted by customer/patient name or by drug name. Sorting and printing the labels by drug name makes the filling task of actually putting the pills in the cassettes much easier. Click on the desired **SORT BY** choice.

Choose *Drug*.

11 Click on the appropriate **PRINT** choice.

Choose *All*.

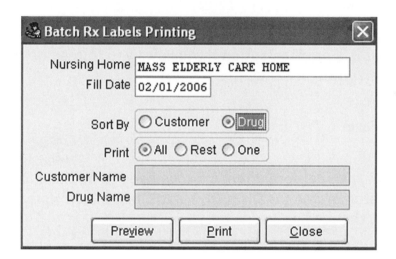

12 Click on **PREVIEW**.

13 After viewing the refill list, click on the **PRINT** icon located at the top of the *Report Designer* menu.

Exercise

1 Following the steps in this lab, print labels to refill medication for Coolidge Corner Nursing Home. Use 04/26/2005 as the refill date. Sort by customer/patient and print for one customer/patient: Floyd Ellis.

2 Print the labels for Floyd Ellis, affix the labels to the appropriate cassettes, and fill the cassettes for Floyd Ellis. Arrange the cassettes and stock bottles for verification. When this exercise is completed, notify your instructor that you are ready for assessment.

Questions for Review

1 Nursing home labels may be sorted by drug name or patient name.

   a True

   b False

2 *Rest* is a printing option that allows you to resume previously interrupted printing.

   a True

   b False

3 How many different medications need to be filled for Kinley B. Abston on the 02/01/2006 Mass Elderly Care Home batch refill? List the medication names.

4 Who is patient Verna Bushey's prescribing physician?

5 What is the sig for patient Sarah King's Xanax?

ASSESSMENT

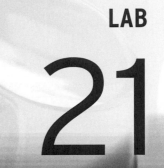

Comprehensive Application Test

Dr. Emma Drive   *office: 800/777-2211*
31252 Phone Street
Gabby, NY 01263

Patient Name:___Catelynn Judith Starr
Date:___9/7/07
Address:_____

    Refill:_____1 Times

    Rx: Tegretol 100mg Chew
        Bid
      #60

Dr. Emma Drive

Product Selection Permitted	Dispense As Written

DEA NO.___AD12352349
Address_____

Enter the prescription above into the pharmacy software database. Use the Assessment Checklist as a guide to the skills that will be evaluated.

DESCRIPTION OF ASSESSMENT	POINTS POSSIBLE	POINTS EARNED/ COMMENTS
Receiving the Retail Prescription		
Student read through the entire prescription before entering information into the database.	**2**	
Using good customer service and communication skills, the student asked the "new customer" all pertinent questions: • Is the customer taking any other medications? Rx, OTC, herbals? • Does the customer have any allergies? • What is the payment source? Insurance, cash? • What is the customer's identifying information? Full name, DOB, address, phone information?	**5**	
Data Entry		
Patient name is entered in correct format (last name, comma, space, first name) and added to the database. All patient information is saved correctly.	**18**	
Family head is entered correctly and added to the database.	**10**	
Prescriber is added to the database and saved correctly.	**10**	
Student's initials are added to the form.	**2**	
New customer is made aware of pharmacy's HIPAA policy and notation is made to customer form.	**3**	
Insurance information is entered correctly.	**5**	
Disease, other drugs, and allergy profiles are updated.	**5**	
Correct medication name, dosage, prescribed quantity, and refills are added. Correct days supply is added. Correct DAW code is selected. Correct prescription date is entered.	**10**	
Correct abbreviated sig is added.	**5**	

Filling the Medication Order

Label is printed. Label is compared and double-checked with
the hard-copy prescription.   **5**

Medication is filled by taking the label to the shelf to   **15**
compare NDC numbers. Medication is counted and put in
appropriate vial. Correct label is affixed to vial and second
part of label is attached to the prescription hard copy.
The prescription is prepared for the pharmacist to check.
Appropriate checks have been made while filling the
prescription order.

Completion

Using customer service skills, customer transaction is   **4**
completed. Counseling is offered, and correct change made.

Stock medication bottle is returned to shelf. Hard copy is filed.   **1**

Totals   **100**

Key for New Customer Information

Customer information:
Phone: 712/777-3434
Date of Birth (DOB): February 25, 1996
Allergies: PCN
Other Meds: Seasonal Singulair 4 mg chewable tablets

PCS

Starr, Dora E   00
Starr, Catelynn J. 02
ID # JK2233669875232
Group# JS236
Rx Bin: 610415
Electronic Processor: 3211203827

Family Head:
Dora E. Starr
24 Guitar Way
Freetown, IA 51206

APPENDIX A
Sig Abbreviation Shortcuts

ABBREVIATION	MEANING
1-2	1 or 2
1-2G	1 or 2 drops
1 APP	1 applicator
1C	1 capsule
1CBID	Take 1 capsule twice each day
1CQD	Take 1 capsule daily
1CQID	Take 1 capsule four times a day
1CTID	Take 1 capsule three times a day
1DR	Take 1 teaspoon
1G	1 drop
1IAPP	Insert 1 applicator
1SSTS	Take 1 ½ teaspoon
1T	1 tablet
1TBID	1 tablet twice a day
1TPOBID	1 tablet by mouth twice a day
1TPOQD	1 tablet by mouth each day
1TPOQDHS	1 tablet by mouth every day at bedtime
1TQD	1 tablet each day
1TQID	1 tablet four times a day
1TTID	1 tablet three times a day
2C	2 capsules
2G	2 drops
2T	2 tablets
3G	3 drops
3TSP	3 teaspoon
4G	4 drops
4HRS	4 hours
AA	Affected area
AAA	Apply to affected area
AAD	After dinner
AAS	After supper
AC	Before meals
AD	As directed
AE	Into the affected eye
AM	Morning

ABBREVIATION	MEANING
AND	And
AP	Apply
BID	Twice a day
BP	Blood pressure
C	With
CAP	Capsule
CCM	With food or milk
CF	With food
CM	With meals
D	Daily
D1T	Dissolve 1 tablet
DA	Dissolve and
DAY	Day
DIA	Diarrhea
DIS	Dissolve
DR	Drink
DWW	Dilute with water
EN	Each nostril
EVERY	Every
F	For
F1	For 1 week
F10	For 10 days
F14	For 14 days
F2	For 2 weeks
F5	For 5 days
F7	For 7 days
FE	For external use only
FIN	Finished
FP	For pain
GTT	Drop
GTTS	Drops
H	Hours
HA	Headache
HOUR	Hour
HS	Bedtime
I	Instill
I1G	Instill 1 drop
I1P	Inhale 1 puff
I1S	Insert 1 suppository
I1T	Insert 1 tablet
I2G	Instill 2 drops
I2P	Inhale 2 puffs
I3G	Instill 3 drops
I3P	Inhale 3 puffs
I4G	Instill 4 drops
I4P	Inhale 4 puffs
I5G	Instill 5 drops
INFECT	Infection
IJ	In juice
IL	In liquids
INF	For infection
INS	Insert

ABBREVIATION	MEANING
ITCH	Itching
IW	In water
L	Left
LE	Left ear
N	Nerves
NV	Nausea and vomitting
OA	Into affected eye
OD	Into right eye
OS	Into left eye
OU	Into both eyes
P	For pain
PIT	Place 1 tablet
PA	Pain
PAC	Packet
PATCH	Patch
PC	After meals
PL	Place
PO	By mouth
PRN	As needed
PRNA	As needed for anxiety
PRNC	As needed for cough
PRND	As needed for diarrhea
PRNF	As needed for
PRNHA	As needed for headache
PRNP	As needed for pain
Q	Every
Q12H	Every 12 hours
Q3-4H	Every 3 to 4 hours
Q4-6H	Every 4 to 6 hours
Q4H	Every 4 hours
Q6-8H	Every 6 to 8 hours
Q6H	Every 6 hours
Q8H	Every 8 hours
QAM	Every morning
QD	Daily
QID	Four times a day
QOD	Every other day
QPM	Every evening
R	Right
RE	Right ear
S	Suppository
S2D	Squirt twice daily
SL	Under tongue
SS	$\frac{1}{2}$
SSAP	$\frac{1}{2}$ applicator
SSTSP	$\frac{1}{2}$ teaspoon
T	Take
T1	Take 1
T1C	Take 1 capsule

ABBREVIATION	MEANING
T1-2C	Take 1 or 2 capsules
T1-2T	Take 1 or 2 tablets
T1SST	Take 1 ½ tablets
TID	Three times a day
T1TBL	Take 1 tablespoonful
T1TBS	Take 1 tablespoonful
T1TSP	Take 1 teaspoonful
T2	Take 2
T2C	Take 2 capsules
T2TSP	Take 2 teaspoons
T2T	Take 2 tablets
T3	Take 3
T3C	Take 3 capsules
T3T	Take 3 tablets
T3TSP	Take 3 teaspoons
T4C	Take 4 capsules
T4T	Take 4 tablets
T4TSP	Take 4 teaspoons
T5C	Take 5 capsules
T5T	Take 5 tablets
TAKE	Take
TBID	Take 1 tablet twice a day
TBL	Tablespoonful
TBSP	Tablespoonful
THEN	Then
TID	Three times a day
TK	Take
TLA	To large area
TSP	Teaspoonful
TSST	Take ½ tablet
TUD	Take as directed
TTSP	Take ½ teaspoonful
U	Until all taken
U2I	Use 2 inhalations
U2P	Use 2 puffs
U2S	Use 2 sprays
UAT	Until all taken
UD	As directed
UF	Until finished
UG	Until gone
USE	Use
UUD	Use as directed
WF	With food
WJ	With juice
WM	With meals
WMB	With meals and bedtime
WW	With water

APPENDIX B
Practice Exercises

Exercise

Answer the questions relating to each prescription sig. Assume that generic substitutions are allowed unless otherwise indicated.

Epivir #60
1 tab po bid

Refill × 6

How many tablets will you dispense?

How many days will the prescription last?

How many refills are permitted?

What is the DAW code?

Print the signa as it should appear on the patient's bottle.

Ampicillin   250 mg   200 ml
1 tsp po qid

Refill x 1

How many milliliters (ml) will you dispense?

How many days will the prescription last?

How many refills are permitted?

What is the DAW code?

Print the signa as it should appear on the patient's bottle.

Ritalin   5 mg #30   (Schedule II medication)
I tab po qAM for ADHD

Daw
Refill 1

How many tablets will you dispense?

How many days will the prescription last?

How many refills are permitted?

What is the DAW code?

Print the signa as it should appear on the patient's bottle.

Dyazide   #30
1 cap po qAM

Brand Name Medically Necessary
Refill x 5

How many capsules will you dispense?

How many days will the prescription last?

How many refills are permitted?

What is the DAW code?

Print the signa as it should appear on the patient's bottle.

Coreg 6.25 mg   #60
1 tab po qAM and qPM

Refill prn

How many tablets will you dispense?

How many days will the prescription last?

How many refills are permitted?

What is the DAW code?

Print the signa as it should appear on the patient's bottle.

Exercise

Write the following sigs correctly by using the sig abbreviation shortcuts.

1 Take 1 tablet by mouth every day

2 Inject 35 units subcutaneously every morning

3 Take 1 to 2 teaspoonfuls by mouth every 6 to 8 hours

4 Instill 5 drops in the left eye two times daily

5 Insert one suppository per rectum every 12 hours as needed for hemorrhoids

Prescription Processing Practice

Exercise

Process the following prescriptions. You may need to add new patient and/or doctor information to the database. Use the blank prescriptions on pages 204 and 205 to create your own exercises. Remember: The DEA numbers will be flagged as invalid.

Dr. Robert Clear
300 Fairfield Street
Newton, MA 02456

office: 617/261-6610
fax: 617/556-2300

Patient Name: Andrew Shedlock
Date: 5/10/2007
Address:_____

    Refill:_____1 Times

    Rx: Amoxicillin 250 mg #30
        I cap pot id on empty stomach

Robert Clear

Product Selection Permitted	Dispense As Written

DEA NO.____AC4382165
Address_____

Dr. Robert Clear
300 Fairfield Street
Newton, MA 02456

office: 617/261-6610
fax: 617/556-2300

Patient Name:__ Mary Shedlock
Date:__ 4/10/2007
Address:_____

    Refill:____ 0 Times

    Rx: Zithromax 250mg   #6
          ii caps stat the I cap po qd x4d

Robert Clear

Product Selection Permitted	Dispense As Written

DEA NO.__ AC4382165_____
Address_____

Dr. Robert Clear
300 Fairfield Street
Newton, MA 02456

office: 617/261-6610
fax: 617/556-2300

Patient Name:__ Jada Sanchez
Date:__ 7/10/2007
Address:_____

    Refill:____ 0 Times

    Rx: Trimox 125mg/5ml   150ml
        I tsp pot id x 10d
        Refrigerate

Robert Clear

Product Selection Permitted	Dispense As Written

DEA NO.__ AC4382165_____
Address_____

Dr. Nathan Goldberg
123 Gold St.
Allston, MA 02134

office: 617/443-3343
fax: 617/645-1500

Patient Name:___Julia Lowther___
Date:___7/10/2007___
Address:_____

    Refill:_____1 Times___

    Rx: APAP/Hydrocodone 7.5mg   #20
       I tab po q 4-6 h prn pain
       may cause drowsiness

Nathan Goldberg

Product Selection Permitted	Dispense As Written

DEA NO._____
Address_____

Dr. Nathan Goldberg
123 Gold St.
Allston, MA 02134

office: 617/443-3343
fax: 617/645-1500

Patient Name:___Patricia Armstrong___
Date:___6/10/2007___
Address:_____

    Refill:_____5 Times___

    Rx: Triphasil 28
       as directed

Nathan Goldberg

Product Selection Permitted	Dispense As Written

DEA NO._____
Address_____

Dr. Nathan Goldberg   *office: 617/443-3343*
123 Gold St.   *fax: 617/645-1500*
Allston, MA 02134

Patient Name:＿＿Patricia Armstrong＿
Date:＿6/10/2007＿
Address:＿＿＿＿＿＿＿＿＿＿＿＿＿＿＿＿＿＿＿＿＿＿＿

      Refill:＿＿＿6 Times＿＿

      Rx: Levothyroxine 0.075mg
           I tap po qam on empty stomach
           #30

Nathan Goldberg

Product Selection Permitted	Dispense As Written

DEA NO.＿＿＿＿＿＿＿＿＿＿＿＿＿
Address＿＿＿＿＿＿＿＿＿＿＿＿＿＿＿＿＿＿＿

Dr. Nathan Goldberg   *office: 617/443-3343*
123 Gold St.   *fax: 617/645-1500*
Allston, MA 02134

Patient Name:＿＿Elzora Banaskey＿
Date:＿8/10/2007＿
Address:＿＿＿＿＿＿＿＿＿＿＿＿＿＿＿＿＿＿＿＿＿＿＿

      Refill:＿＿＿1 Times＿＿

      Rx: Augumentin 250mg/5ml
           i tsp po q 8h x 10d
           150ml
           take with yogurt, refrigerate

Nathan Goldberg

Product Selection Permitted	Dispense As Written

DEA NO.＿＿＿＿＿＿＿＿＿＿＿＿＿
Address＿＿＿＿＿＿＿＿＿＿＿＿＿＿＿＿＿＿＿

Dr. Stephen Hardy
76 Walnut St.
Allston, MA 02134

office: 617/532-6390
fax: 617/435-6300

Patient Name:___Annie Morris___
Date:___4/12/2007___
Address:_____

     Refill:_____0 Times_

     Rx: amoxicillin 250mg
          I tsp po q 8h x 10d
          #150ml

Steve Hardy

Product Selection Permitted   Dispense As Written

DEA NO. AH4442149RES___
Address_____

Dr. Stephen Hardy
76 Walnut St.
Allston, MA 02134

office: 617/532-6390
fax: 617/435-6300

Patient Name:___Stephanie Richards___
Date:___4/12/2007___
Address:_____

     Refill:_____5 Times_

     Rx: Ambien 10mg
          I tap po hs
          #30

Steve Hardy

Product Selection Permitted   Dispense As Written

DEA NO. AH4442149RES_____
Address_____

Dr. Stephen Hardy
76 Walnut St.
Allston, MA 02134

office: 617/532-6390
fax: 617/435-6300

Patient Name:___Stephanie Richards
Date:___4/12/2007
Address:_____

Refill:_____0 Times

Rx: Cortisporin Otic Suspension
v gtts ad q 4-6h prn infection
7.5ml

Steve Hardy

Product Selection Permitted	Dispense As Written

DEA NO. _AH4442149RES__
Address_____

Patient Name:_____
Date:_____
Address _____

Refill:_____Times

Rx:

Product Selection Permitted	Dispense As Written

DEA NO. _____
Address_____

Patient Name:_____

Date:_____

Address _____

      Refill:_____Times

      Rx:

Product Selection Permitted   Dispense As Written

DEA NO. _____

Address_____